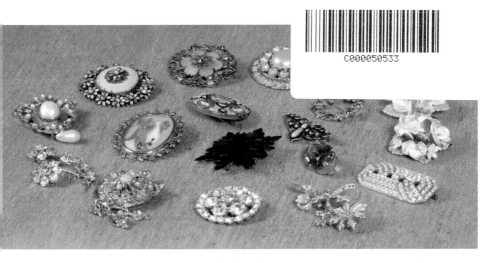

A collection of costume-jewellery brooches, fashionable between the two world wars. Several are reproductions of styles from other periods. Pearls, paste and coloured glass stones are used with small turquoises in the floral spray example (bottom right). The two floral ones (far right) are delicate Staffordshire pottery flowers; the black one (centre) is French jet; the dog's head (left of the French jet) has been hand-embroidered and mounted in silver metal; and there are two Italian mosaic examples (one above the French jet and the other top right). The small butterfly (right of the French jet) is set with turquoises and pink stones on a mother-of-pearl base with green and blue enamel.

Ladies' Dress Accessories

Eleanor Johnson

A Shire book

Published in 2004 by Shire Publications Ltd,
Cromwell House, Church Street, Princes Risborough,
Buckinghamshire HP27 9AA, UK.
(Website: www.shirebooks.co.uk)

British Library Cataloguing in Publication Data:
Johnson, Eleanor.
Ladies' dress accessories. – (Shire album; 421)
1. Dress accessories – History
2. Dress accessories – Collectors and collecting
I. Title 391.4'4
ISBN 0 7478 0570 9

Cover: *A selection of the items featured in this book. (Left, from top to bottom) Gilt-metal chain purse; mother-of-pearl buckle; silver Art Nouveau brooch; 'Conway' souvenir purse. (Centre row) Gold bracelet; 'Mischief' perfume in a well-known bottle; gold 'Durham Light Infantry' brooch; photograph showing the type of dress typical of the Edwardian period, covered in this book; buttonhook with mother-of-pearl handle; black glass earrings; silver-handled buttonhook. (Right-hand row) Brass skirt lifter; gilt chain with typical Art Deco square pendant. (Right) Two hatpins with decorative tops.*

ACKNOWLEDGEMENTS
The author would like to acknowledge with gratitude her thanks for the loan of items for the photographs and for actual photographs to: Kathleen Alcock; Jennifer Allen; Toni Batcheldor; Lorraine Bean; Audrey Blofield; Edith Cansdale; Margery Cutbush; Elaine Gaussen; Doreen Gretton; Marion Howitt; Dee McCoull of R. A. Dyer, Ilminster; Rosemary Moore; Jean Mott; Delia Pearmund; Mary Rendell; Janet Singleton; Val and Francis Watson; Joyce Westwood; Sue Willows; and also to the trustees of the Cavalcade of Costume, Lime Tree House, Blandford Forum, Dorset, for the two specially taken photographs on pages 32 (bottom) and 39. Michael Bass took the photographs on pages 9 (bottom), 13, 14, 44 (bottom), 45 (lower), 48 and 52. Other modern photographs are by David A. Ross LRPS.

Printed in Malta by Gutenberg Press Limited, Gudja Road,
Tarxien PLA 19, Malta.

Contents

Introduction 4
The dressing table and dressing accessories 7
Scent bottles 13
Jewellery 18
Buttons and buckles 26
Buttonhooks and shoehorns 29
Hatpins and hatpin holders 32
Gloves, glove stretchers, powdering flasks
    and glove boxes 36
Skirt lifters 38
Handbags, purses and chatelaines 39
Spectacles, quizzing glasses and lorgnettes 44
Card cases, aides-mémoire and notebooks 46
Posy holders 48
Fans 49
Parasols 52
Further reading 53
Places to visit 54
Index 56

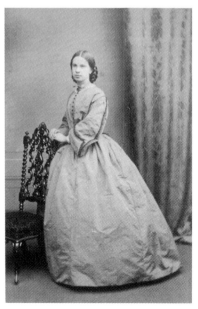

A lady in a crinoline dress with wide sleeves, the bodice buttoned from high neck to waist, probably around the middle of the nineteenth century.

3

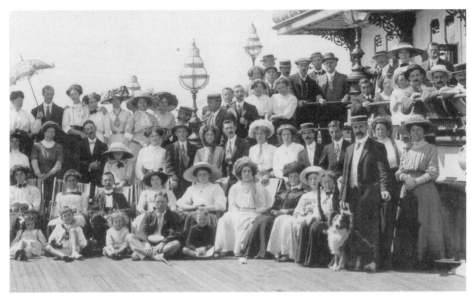

An Edwardian sea-front group, showing the typical dress and hats of the period.

Introduction

Dress accessories have always developed alongside styles of actual dress. Women have wanted to look attractive and changes in fashion have reflected this. Although styles at any one period do not necessarily attract women living in later times, revivals of former ideas do often appear in the work of couture producers, and the high fashions of couture are eventually adopted by a wider clientele. Fashion also reflects variations in social position, age and individual personality. In the nineteenth century there were strict codes of behaviour and dress, and, while criticising any diversion from what was expected in society, women also wanted to stand out among their contemporaries. Another factor that influenced women's dress style was social standing and wealth: many men in the growing industrial fields became much better off financially and wanted their wives to reflect their new status, so dress became more elaborate and often used more varied and costly materials. This trend applied especially to jewellery, but also to other accessories.

In the nineteenth century fashions changed much more rapidly than hitherto, with many confused influences and styles. The growth of new industrial processes, easier domestic and foreign travel and increasing migration from the country to the towns all played a part, making available and simplifying the purchase of a wider variety of materials and accessories, many of which were imported from abroad. The growing prosperity of the middle classes (at its peak in the 1870s), the introduction of mass production, the appearance of the first department stores and the invention of the chain-stitch sewing machine were important influences.

In the early part of the nineteenth century, upper- and middle-class women had solely been expected to be charming and attractive and to be occupied with the accepted feminine activities and accomplishments, leaving the servants to be responsible for domestic chores, but as the years passed women began to revolt against these attitudes and sought greater emancipation, especially after the end of the First World War in 1918. During the 1850s it had become fashionable to drive or stroll in the public parks and gardens, showing off one's latest ensemble and admiring or criticising those of other ladies in the parade.

Following the death of Queen Victoria and her succession by King Edward VII, there were further great changes. After the rather sombre and colourless lifestyle that had followed the death of Prince Albert, and the subsequent mourning of the Queen, life began to change even further, rapidly becoming freer, gayer and brighter. This change was reflected in the style of behaviour and dress of the people, which continued until the outbreak of the Second World War, when, once again, life was forced to change. There was complete concentration on the war effort until, at length, peace brought a slower return to normality, with the eventual end of rationing – of clothes as well as other

A late Victorian postcard showing the typical dress of the period.

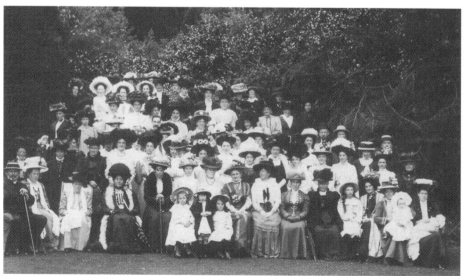

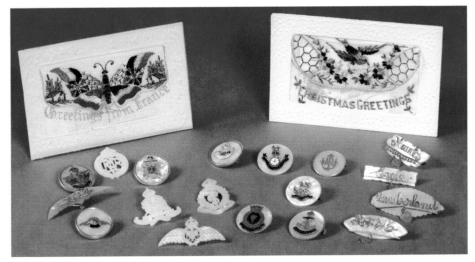

A collection of Royal Navy, Army and Air Force mother-of-pearl sweetheart brooches, photographed with two embroidered cards from the First World War. Several of the brooches are carved from solid shell and others are mounted in silver metal; the badges are of gilt metal with additional painted colour. The three at the top of the column at far right have the names of warships in brass, with small gilt hearts suspended; the similar one bottom right is RASC (Royal Army Service Corps).

necessaries – so that fashion and a wide variety of accessories once more became acceptable, and more free and easy styles became the norm, widening the present-day possibilities for the collecting of dress accessories.

This book is concerned with dress accessories from the middle of the nineteenth century to the end of the Second World War in 1945, when life again changed dramatically in so many ways after the wartime lull in fashion interest, when many women were in uniform in the armed services and there were few accessories.

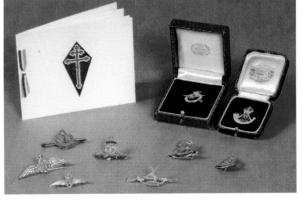

A collection of Royal Navy, Army and Air Force souvenir brooches photographed with a Second World War 'Free France' (France Libre) Christmas card, hand-painted with the Cross of Lorraine and finished with a red, white and blue ribbon. It was printed by Raphael Tuck & Sons for 'Forces Françaises Libres'. All the brooches are from the Second World War except for the gold rifle-shaped one in the centre, which is from the First World War. The two brooches of the Royal Air Force and the one of the Royal Artillery are silver; the naval bar brooch (top left) and The Queen's Royal Regiment and Royal Army Medical Corps brooches (top right) are of silver-coloured metal. The Royal Air Force brooch in the box on the left is hallmarked gold, as is The Durham Light Infantry one on the right. The boxes are those in which the brooches were sold, and bear the names of the jewellers on the silk lining of the lids.

The dressing table and dressing accessories

The dressing table was most important to every self-respecting lady as she dressed and groomed herself, applied her make-up and prepared to go out – a very different approach from the increasingly casual attitude of women since the Second World War and on into the twenty-first century. On this table she would have her hand mirror, hairbrush, comb and clothes brush, many of these in matching sets, together with a variety of small boxes made of silver, porcelain, ivory, wood or enamel. Most of the enamel boxes were made in Staffordshire, particularly at Bilston, or at Battersea in London. Glass boxes, bottles and pots with silver tops and those of English or French porcelain were

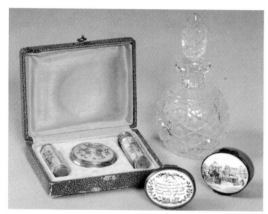

also popular. Some, which were curved inside, were used for creams or rouge, and others contained comfits or cachous (to sweeten the breath).

Left: (Left) A fine-quality early-twentieth-century make-up set in a fitted box, containing lipstick, powder compact and perfume atomiser. (Back right) A heavy cut-glass scent bottle with ornate stopper. (Front) Two patch boxes, the one on the left being of Battersea or Bilston enamel on copper and bearing a message; the one on the right being of green porcelain and decorated with a coloured period scene.

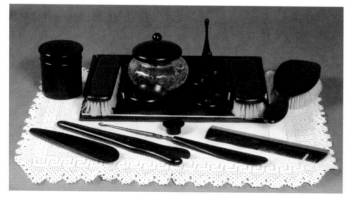

A complete ebony dressing-table set with tray comprising, to the right of the tray, a hairbrush, and, on the tray, two clothes brushes, a lidded powder bowl, two ring stands, a shallow stud tray and a small rouge pot. To the left of the tray is a hair tidy. In front, from left to right, are a shoehorn, a pair of glove stretchers, a combined shoe buttonhook and shoehorn, and a silver-backed comb. The set is photographed on a linen hand-crochet-edged tray cloth.

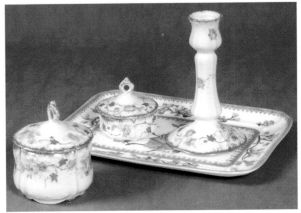

Four typical dressing-table-set items in floral-decorated china. The tray is in Royal Worcester porcelain of the late nineteenth century, and the candlestick, lidded powder bowl and trinket pot are Limoges china of a slightly later period.

Many of the items used by nineteenth-century ladies as they dressed appeal to collectors. Elaborate hairstyles needed hair combs; these consisted of a number of gently curved prongs made of pressed-out silver, some other metal or tortoiseshell with a fancy heading, some set with foil-backed paste jewels or semi-precious stones. Silver filigree and scrollwork patterns were popular, followed by a passion for Eastern designs, with Islamic motifs, looped chains and imitation stones of coloured glass. Cut-steel decoration was popular during the middle years of the century and was often used to ornament tortoiseshell combs, as was piqué, which is an inlay of small silver or gold dots. More elaborate inlays, called posé, used sheet gold or silver. Other ideas in the form of cameos, mosaic and coral were obtained from the Continent or further afield. During the 1860s it became fashionable to wear the hair in a chignon or coarse net, and large ornate combs fastened this to the main hair. In 1861 the death of her husband plunged Queen Victoria and her court into mourning, and black hair combs appeared to match the appropriate dress and jewellery. Most of these were made of real English jet from Whitby or of so-called French jet – actually black glass cut and set to simulate the real thing. In the late nineteenth and early twentieth century, silver combs became popular, some set with semi-precious stones or in the naturalistic and flowing Art Nouveau

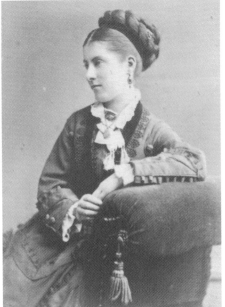

A lady with a built-up, padded hairstyle and lacy fichu at the neck, secured with a large brooch, probably late nineteenth century.

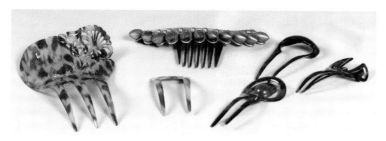

A group of hair combs. At the back is an elaborate Edwardian heavy crescent with engraved gilt pointed decorations, small and larger balls, and a central, hinged black plastic comb. The remainder, all of imitation tortoiseshell, are from the early twentieth century, the large one on the left having a pierced decoration.

A group of Edwardian mother-of-pearl hair combs. The one at the top left has an imitation-tortoiseshell comb.

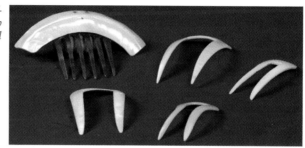

designs initiated by William Morris and his followers.

Seated at her dressing table, a lady would dress her hair or have it dressed by her personal maid, using the combs to secure the elaborate coiffure in place. She would proceed to apply her make-up and perfume and select and put on her rings from her ring stand and other jewellery from a specially fitted jewellery

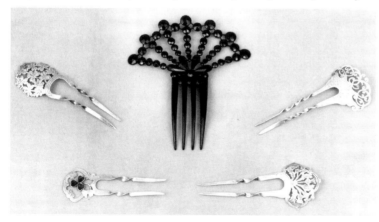

Hair combs. (Top row from left) Silver with trefoil design; French jet in fan design; engraved scrolled silver, dated 1897. (Bottom row) Silver with chrysoprase trefoil inset, dated 1905; silver with thistle design, dated 1906.

9

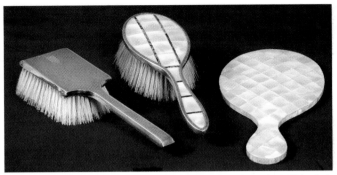

Three dressing-table items. (Left) A silver-backed hairbrush, hallmarked, assayed in Birmingham in 1938. The hallmark gives a symbol for the office in which the item was assayed and a date letter, together with a mark proving the purity of the silver and often a maker's mark. (Centre and right) A mother-of-pearl-backed hairbrush and hand mirror.

Four buttonhole holders. (Top, left to right) Two brass ones, each with a clip to secure the holder; a delicate glass one with a glass hook. (Bottom) A decorative silver example with a brooch pin.

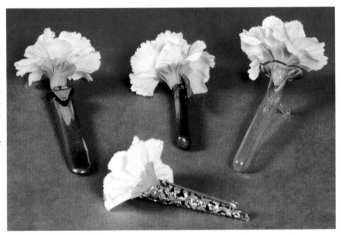

A group of dress clips, 1920s and 1930s. (Above, left to right) A mother-of-pearl matching pair; two single shell flower shapes; a single amber-coloured plastic clip with a diamanté-studded strip down the centre; a single mother-of-pearl leaf shape. (Below, left to right) A single shell butterfly shape; a matching heart-shaped pair set with turquoises; a single deeply carved mother-of-pearl clip.

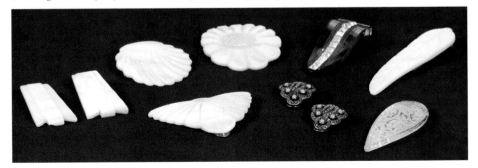

An elaborate yellow-beaded girdle with beaded tassels, and a porcelain scarf ring painted with a yellow rose and set in a silver mount. Below it, a cloak chain with silver leaves.

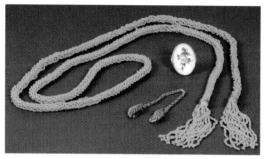

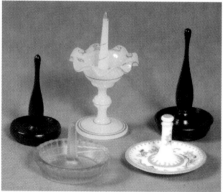

A collection of ring stands. (Left to right) Ebony; glass; unusual gilt-decorated elaborately shaped opaline glass; floral-decorated Royal Worcester porcelain; and another, larger, ebony example.

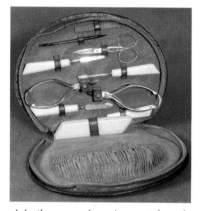

A leather-covered manicure set from the early 1940s, closed with a zip-fastener, containing a comprehensive complement of fingernail necessities.

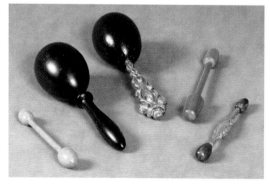

A group of darners. (Left to right) Small boxwood glove darner; plain ebony; ebony with a silver handle; a plain wood glove darner; another glove darner, having a silver handle with green-painted ends.

box. Having then put on her shoes or boots with the help of a buttonhook and shoehorn, she would array herself in her chosen costume and put on her hat, which would be secured with hatpins. Her gloves would then be put on, perhaps again with the help of a buttonhook, and she was ready to take up the things she needed to carry – a chatelaine, or a handbag or purse into

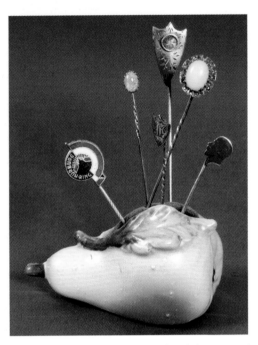

A small collection of tie or stick pins, displayed in a pear-shaped china pincushion. (Left to right) Green, white and black enamel with the lettering 'NURBURG RING' (possibly a continental souvenir); an opal set in gold; a small engraved shield, which may have held a stone; another, smaller, engraved shield; a moonstone set in a gilt mount with marcasite; and a silver head, possibly depicting King George V.

which she would put her lorgnette or spectacles and a card case. Lastly she would take up her fan, and maybe a posy holder or a parasol.

Ring stands are collectable items. They provided a useful means of keeping safe precious, easily mislaid rings. They are usually formed like the branch of a tree, or like a hand with the fingers extended, on a base, although some consist of a central rod or cone, with or without hooks. They were made in silver, silver plate, ivory, wood, glass, china or pottery, including Wedgwood Jasper ware, which has a matt finish to the raised motif in white on a coloured ground.

Also to be found are manicure sets and tools.

Scent bottles

Perfume has a long and fascinating history, being used on the person as well as having a ritual and religious significance since very early times. It was always a luxury commodity and early containers were made in costly materials to be worthy of their expensive contents. Sweet-scented substances were used in creams and ointments for use on the skin, produced in solid form to be carried in pomanders and used for smelling salts, also in concentrated form or in toilet waters. It is these specific uses that produced such variety in the containers which interest present-day collectors. In more modern times the sole use of perfume has been to make women more attractive, but in former days it was believed it could prevent infection and also served – particularly

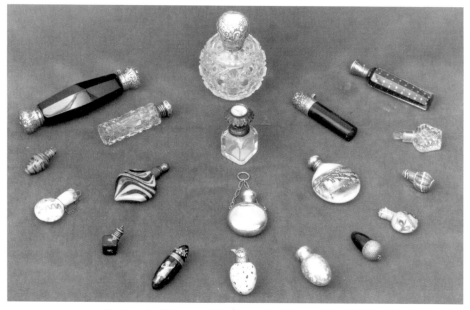

Scent bottles. (Lower ring from left) Three small late-nineteenth-century Venetian glass bottles made for the tourist trade, each with its original stopper, one green, one white with coloured decoration, and a small dark green one shaped like a die; dark red enamel torpedo shape decorated with a figure, with flowers on the hinged lid, and with silver gilt mounts; porcelain egg with silver bird head for the top; silver egg shape with finely chased decoration; acorn shape in deep ruby glass, with gilt cup; two more in Venetian glass; small bottle in moulded glass with matching stopper. (Inner ring from left) Deep blue glass double-ended type with silver mounts and lids; small cylindrical cut glass with silver screw top; flat multicoloured and silvered glass with tight-fitting stopper, Italian, of the nineteenth and twentieth centuries; flat silver chatelaine bottle; porcelain with transfer print of Prestatyn pier and silver top; deep ruby glass with finely chased hinged silver top; clear glass lined with deep blue, decorated with gold stars and having a hinged gold top. (Top centre) Heavy round cut-glass dressing-table cologne bottle with silver screw top. (Below this) Square clear-glass bottle with lithograph print set in lid.

in crowded theatres and ill-ventilated ballrooms – to mask the results of the inability to easily clean elaborate dress. Most ladies made their own perfumes or had them made for them personally, supplied in plain bottles, the contents of which they then decanted into their own more decorative containers.

There was a huge growth in the perfume industry at the beginning of the nineteenth century, and as the century progressed industrial expansion brought greater affluence to a much wider range of the population and better industrial processes made perfume available to a larger public. Numerous varied scent bottles were produced in the nineteenth century; a great many were made of cut decorative clear glass with silver tops, for cologne or lavender water, but as in other fields ingenuity and imagination in design, together with the use of new materials and a wide range of skills, produced an extensive choice. To a large extent, the very nature of scent has governed the design of its containers. The fact that it is so volatile necessitates a tight-fitting lid, and protection from strong light is sometimes important to prevent deterioration.

Scent bottles could be made of porcelain of either English or continental origin, and some well-known English firms such as Wedgwood, Spode, Derby, Coalport and the Worcester Royal Porcelain Company produced decorative and attractive bottles. In the latter part of the nineteenth century large numbers of relatively inexpensive containers were made in the Staffordshire Potteries. Glass was also frequently used, much from English factories at Stourbridge, Nailsea and Bristol, and there were some very attractive types, including Opaline, Venetian, Cameo, Aventurine and a type enamelled with trailed patterns. Another kind was overlay, in which a layer of coloured glass was fused

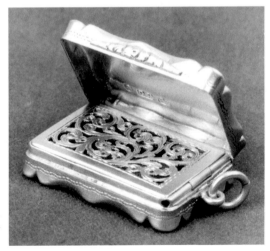

A very fine example of a silver vinaigrette, with the original gilded grille in elaborate scrollwork. The base and lid are finely engraved.

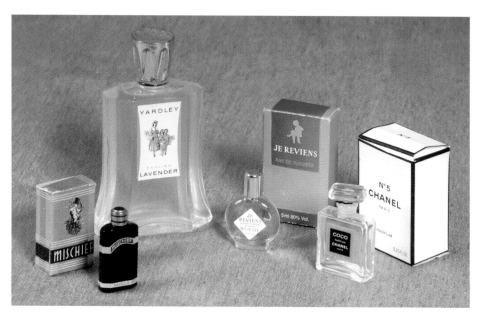

A group of scent bottles from around the 1930s, all but the Yardley Lavender toilet water photographed with their original packaging. 'Mischief', made by Saville (left); 'Je Reviens', made by Worth of Paris (centre); and 'Chanel No. 5' (right), labelled 'Coco, Paris'.

over plain glass and then patterns were cut through the layers with a wheel. Although coloured glass could be used in many forms, one distinctive style was the double-ended container, usually deep blue, red or green. This consisted of two bottles fused together at their bases, one for perfume, with a stopper beneath the lid, and one for smelling salts, with a patent seal inside the lid. Other materials used in the manufacture of perfume bottles included silver, enamel, brass, hardstones, ivory and fruit stones.

Smelling bottles, boxes and vinaigrettes are also perfume related. Vinaigrettes are very small gold or silver boxes, engraved or engine-turned, with a tight-fitting hinged lid to avoid evaporation, and having a perforated grille inside that encloses a small sponge soaked in aromatic vinegar. The inside of the box is heavily gilded to prevent corrosion.

The growth of tourism led to the production of many souvenirs, and these included scent bottles. After the First World War life became very different; women sought more freedom and fun after the conventional and restrictive life of the Victorians – a change that had already begun to take place during the Edwardian period, when women had given up restrictive corsets, started to wear shorter skirts and had their hair cut short. Wearing make-up and using scent in public

15

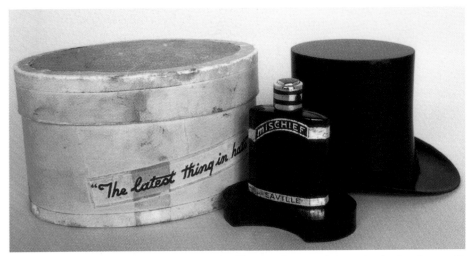

Novelty packaging for 'Mischief' perfume by Saville: a top-hat containing a bottle of perfume, with a hatbox.

became the norm (and drinking and smoking also became acceptable for women), and so the perfume industry expanded. At the beginning of the twentieth century there was a great emphasis on cheaper packaging and presentation. Bakelite, a

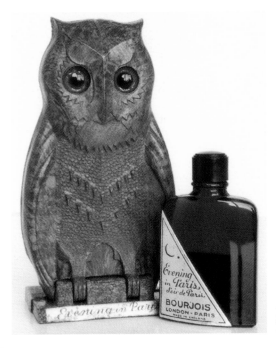

Novelty packaging for 'Evening in Paris' perfume by Bourjois: a plastic owl containing the bottle.

This small poster advertises 'Evening in Paris' perfume by Bourjois, apparently produced as a Royal Jubilee souvenir.

synthetic resin made of a combination of chemicals, was introduced in 1907. Many new perfumiers emerged who later became household names, such as Coty in 1920 with their 'L'Aimant'. Guerlain was another well-known brand, and 'Chanel No. 5' was introduced in 1921, followed in the 1930s by 'Mischief', 'Evening in Paris' and 'Chypre' in novelty-shaped bottles and packaging. The well-known firm of Yardley was established originally in 1775. Some couturiers began to sell perfume in association with their clothes, and this became a growing practice. Also in the 1920s and 1930s huge numbers of bottles in the Art Deco style, so distinctive of the period, in clear and frosted glass and pale colours, were imported from Czechoslovakia, which had become a skilled and prominent producer of glass. The huge demand for perfumes and cosmetics in this period was thus satisfied but was soon to be halted by the onset of the Second World War, during which only the most basic products were available.

Jewellery

The primary purposes of jewellery are to make women appear more attractive and to attract attention. During the nineteenth century clothing fashions and hairstyles changed rapidly, some styles being very short-lived. After the middle years of the century society women were eager to discover and wear the latest, most sensational and novel designs, and the demand for large showy jewellery grew. Those involved in the advancement of new industrial processes and mechanical mass production were only too eager to satisfy this demand, which was also exploited to the full by artists and other craftsmen who were able to make use of the new developments and innovations in production. Gold had for a long time been scarce, leading to the remaking of many pieces of jewellery, but in the nineteenth century the supply became more plentiful when gold was discovered firstly in North America and later in Australia and 'gold rushes' ensued. Another reason for this increased demand as the century progressed was that the middle classes became much better off and more women were able to acquire and to wear jewellery. High-quality and expensive jewellery was more and more being worn by the wives of the new industrialists, their husbands seeing that this was an excellent way of drawing attention to their own position and wealth. But there was a period late in the century when women tended to give up wearing jewellery because it was seen as symbolising a bond, existing because on marriage women became completely subject to their husbands, and jewellery was designed and bought by

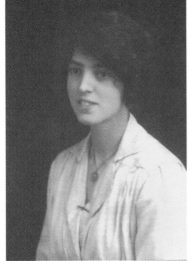

men – so it was not surprising that, at a time when the women's emancipation movement was widening and gathering pace, women began to see jewellery as a symbol of their increasingly resented position and as emphasising the status of men, and so many chose not to wear it.

But jewellery was not out of favour for long. The constant succession of new fashions in garments was matched by changes in popular jewellery. At the more expensive levels of the

A photograph from about 1919 of Mabel Smith wearing a locket on a chain and a bar brooch, possibly one of those displayed in the collection of jewellery in her open leather jewel case shown on the opposite page.

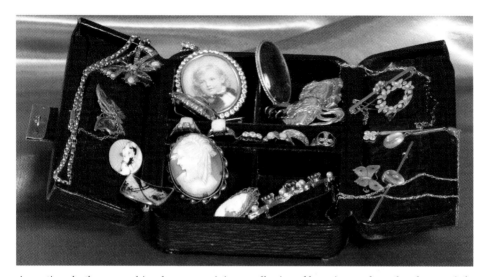

An antique leather-covered jewel case containing a collection of late-nineteenth- and early-twentieth-century jewellery. (Left, top to bottom) A butterfly brooch set with turquoises, rubies and marcasite; another butterfly brooch, mother-of-pearl with turquoises, pink stones and green and blue enamel; two Norwegian enamel-on-silver brooches with Arctic snow scenes, 1906 and 1915. (Centre of case, top, left to right) An exquisite oval gold pendant, set with paste stones, containing a colour-tinted photograph of a young Victorian boy (there is another colour-tinted photograph of this boy's son as a child in the back), and with a heavy gold chain draped over the left side of the case; in front on its side is an elaborate gold brooch with a compartment for hair in the back; an oval butterfly-wing brooch; a diamond-shaped butterfly-wing pendant; in front is a silver brooch of Art Nouveau design. (Across the centre in the ring slot, left to right) A collection of rings: two gold set with opals; gold with three diamonds; Victorian engagement ring, gold with two opals and small emeralds; gold eternity ring set with diamonds; gold Victorian mourning ring, onyx background with a gold cross set with a small onyx central stone and marcasites. (Centre of case, bottom, left to right) A large and a smaller cameo brooch; a brooch set with red and blue glass stones and pearls. (Right, top to bottom) A gold bar brooch set with four seed pearls in the centre; a gold wreath-shaped brooch, leaves set with turquoises and pearls; a delicate gold necklet, with four diamonds at the bottom of a gold strip topped with a diamond and gold chain; a necklet ending in a gold-mounted moonstone; a blue enamel butterfly; a gold bar brooch with a moonstone.

market, gold, silver, platinum and precious gems were much in evidence, but semi-precious stones also became widely used, such as ivory, seed pearls, coral and turquoise, as well as horsehair and Scottish stones; opals too were extremely popular. In addition less expensive metals were used for settings, such as gilt and pinchbeck.

Pearls and diamonds were popular for engagement rings; lockets were made of gold, silver and jet. Cameos and pendants with crosses were also popular, as were designs that featured a cross and heart, symbolising Faith, Hope and Charity. Much valued too were flowers, especially forget-me-nots, as well as insects, butterflies, horseshoes, buckles, shells and stars. When the Eastern influence was at its height, gold knobs and tassels

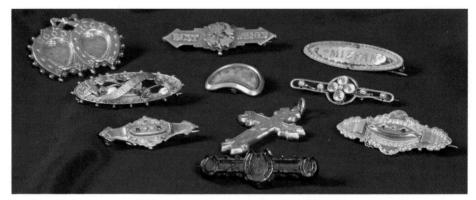

A collection of Victorian and Edwardian gold, gilt and silver brooches and a cross, together with one in bog-oak with a central large carved horseshoe and two smaller horseshoes at the ends. (Left, top to bottom) Gilt pair of hearts with 'GOOD LUCK' surmounted with a bow; gilt 'MIZPAH'; hallmarked gold set with two small garnets. (Centre, top to bottom) Silver with 'BEST WISHES' and a spray of gold leaves in the centre; small gold kidney shape with butterfly-wing decoration; engraved gilt cross with Victorian registration mark on the back. (Right top to bottom) Oval gilt 'MIZPAH'; gold bar brooch set with four round peridots in the centre and four small pearls at the sides; elaborate gold set with two small sapphires.

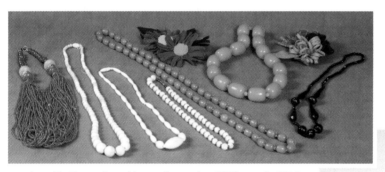

A collection of necklaces from the 1920s and 1930s, photographed with two typical hand-made felt buttonhole decorations. (Left to right) A heavy choker, rows of small coral beads joined to larger coral-coloured and yellow beads below the fastener; ivory; mother-of-pearl; ivory; two of faux amber; black French jet.

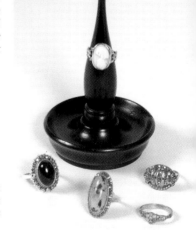

An ebony ring stand, four large rings from the 1920s with artificial stones in decorative settings, and (bottom right) a small mid-twentieth-century solid-gold ring set with turquoises in a flower shape.

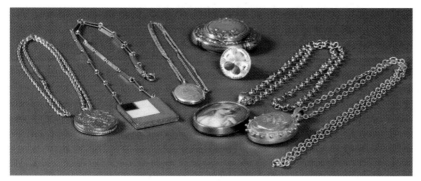

A collection of necklets and lockets with chains, and (top centre) a silver chatelaine patchbox with enclosed mirror in the lid and (below it) a porcelain fob with a hand-painted pansy decoration, the loop for hanging obscured. (Remainder, left to right) An elaborate Victorian engraved gold locket on a gold chain; a square red, cream and black enamel Art Deco pendant on an elaborate gilt chain; a round silver locket containing hair; a miniature painting set in a gold locket with a rolled gold chain, 1840; a heavy silver oval locket and chain with butterfly-wing decoration.

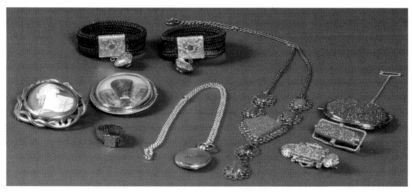

A collection of late Victorian and Edwardian hair and goldstone jewellery. (Left) A gilt-mounted swivel cameo brooch with space for hair in the back. (Top left) A pair of plaited hair bracelets with gilt fastenings and suspended hearts. (Bottom, left to right) A brooch with Prince of Wales feather design in hair; a plaited hair ring with a gold shield for initials; a locket enclosing hair on a gold chain; a gilt necklace set with shaped goldstones; three variously shaped brooches set with goldstones.

were often used and, when Queen Victoria became Empress of India in 1876, many traditional Indian designs were introduced and became fashionable. Mourning and love jewellery in cut steel, Berlin ironwork, ivory, tortoiseshell, onyx, amethyst, pearls and jet had a great vogue, although later they became hated and rejected. Czechoslovakia had become renowned for glass-making, and from the middle of the nineteenth century considerable numbers of artificial stones were made there and exported, including imitation coral, amethyst and turquoise.

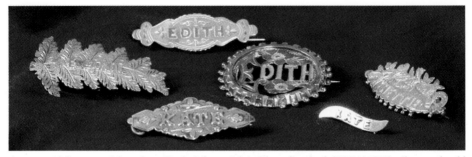

A group of five named brooches. (Back, left to right) Silver fern leaf, 'ELEANOR'; silver and gold 'EDITH'; silver 'EDITH', dated 1882; silver 'HETTIE'. (Front, left to right) Silver 'KATE'; miniature gold 'KATE'.

At this time too, as a result of the increased travel made possible by the coming of the railways, there was a great demand for souvenirs, to which manufacturing jewellers were only too ready to respond, and it was to this end that a proportion of the period's jewellery was produced. Many cheaper mass-produced lockets and brooches were made and in the late 1880s crescent brooches, often using inexpensive moonstones, were popular, as were star designs; also bar and named brooches continued much in favour until the beginning of the twentieth century.

A large number of butterfly brooches particularly date from the 1890s. Pendants set with pink tourmalines or aquamarine were also popular, and peridots were another special favourite. Jewellery featuring the inscription MIZPAH had a great vogue; alluding to Genesis 31:49, 'May the Lord watch between thee and me when we are absent from one another', this refers to the biblical story of Jacob and his brothers, who set up a stone cairn as a sign of their covenant with God. Lockets, rings and brooches bearing this inscription were given when close relations or lovers were about to be parted, for instance by war. Peacock designs were popular in the last quarter of the nineteenth century, and

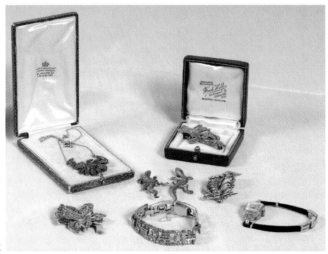

A collection of jewellery featuring marcasite. (Top, left to right) An edelweiss with two leaves, set in silver with a fine chain, presented in its original supplier's box, The London Jeweller's Company, 131 Regent Street, London; a flower spray, set in silver, also in its original jeweller's box, Fred Hill of 99 Regent Street, London. Both are from the late 1930s. (Centre) Two salamander brooches with ruby eyes and a flower spray brooch. (Bottom, left to right) A leaf-shaped brooch; a sectioned bracelet; a marcasite-decorated watch with a black silk wristband.

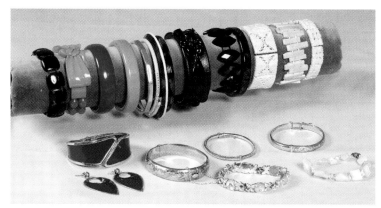

A collection of bracelets from the 1920s, 1930s and 1940s. (On the roll, left to right) Square imitation tortoiseshell sections on elastic; faux amber with bow-shaped decoration; one red and one yellow Bakelite; slim gilt; pink Bakelite inlaid with very small shiny stones; imitation tortoiseshell with cream plastic insert; plain imitation tortoiseshell; two black Bakelite; elliptical-shaped black French jet beads on elastic; imitation tortoiseshell; and three carved bone examples on elastic. Several of these would have been worn above the elbow. (Front, left to right) An Art Deco parure of bracelet and earrings, blue enamel on gilt metal; engraved silver with gold birds and a patent fastening; very slim gold; Trifari pale blue glass stones set in silver metal; gold with a patent fastening; mother-of-pearl sections and beads with a screw fastening.

once again long chains for watches or lorgnettes reappeared. There was a revival of a design in brooches and pendants featuring two hearts or linked rings. There were also good-luck charms, with a shamrock, horseshoes, four-leaf clover or 'Good Luck' inscription, particularly during the Edwardian period (which extended slightly beyond the years of the actual reign of King Edward VII), a time of much gaiety, exuberance and display. Jewellery was being much more widely worn and there was a widespread use of diamanté and paste in imitation of real stones. Marcasite, cut from iron pyrites, was also much in evidence. Costume jewellery became popular, and from the 1890s to 1939 Czechoslovakia produced a distinctive type of such jewellery. In the United States between 1912 and 1917 a firm

A collection of necklaces. (Clockwise from left) Dark ruby-red beads on knotted thread, 1930s; round coral and mother-of-pearl beads; a bracelet and necklace made from small natural pieces of coral; red beads encased in metal mounts separated by pearl beads, 1900 to 1920; imitation blue beads with pearls and gold beads; long rope of simulated-jet beads; mother-of-pearl; graduated cut crystal. (Centre) A typical Art Deco choker of black, red and gold shaped sections on a black-beaded chain.

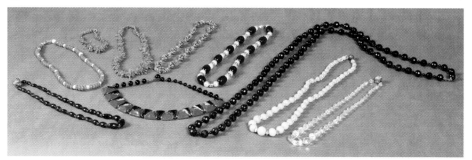

23

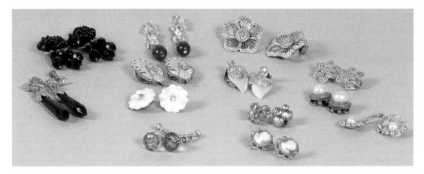

A collection of earrings from the 1920s, 1930s and 1940s. (Left, top to bottom) French jet; black glass droplets mounted in gilt metal with screw fittings. (Second column, top to bottom) Red glass droplets with paste stones in silver-metal mounts and with clip fittings, typical of the 1920s; silver-metal ornate peacocks with clip fittings; mother-of-pearl flower shape; blue glass with screw fittings. (Third column, top to bottom) Large metal five-petalled flower shape; mother-of-pearl and silver metal; pink cut-glass trefoil set in gilt metal with clip fittings; cameos with clip fittings. (Right, top to bottom) Silver-metal six-petalled flower shape set with marcasite; large pearls in marcasite-set surround with clip fitting; small pearls in marcasite-set surround, for pierced ears.

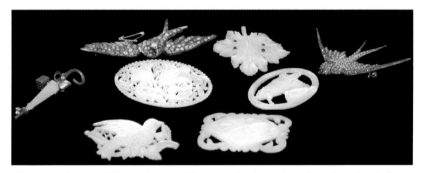

A collection of brooches from the 1920s and 1930s. Six are made of carved mother-of-pearl including a horse's head, a bird and a shaped leaf; the flower holder (far left) is unusual. The two swallows (top left and right) are set with turquoises.

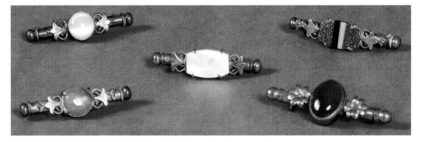

Five 'nanny' or 'sewing' brooches, so called because the central bar contains a slim metal cylinder holding black and white cotton, with needles inside. One end of the bar unscrews to remove the cylinder. These brooches are set with: a moonstone (top left); a yellow stone (bottom left); mother-of-pearl (centre), probably a replacement for the original more common goldstone; goldstone with black and white onyx (top right); an oval amber-coloured stone (bottom right).

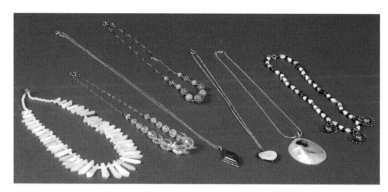

A collection of necklaces and necklets from the 1920s and 1930s. (Left to right) Mother-of-pearl; rhinestones; blue raised butterfly-wing diamond shape on a fine chain; elaborate green and yellow beads; mother-of-pearl heart mounted in silver; mother-of-pearl shell on a fine chain; green and white beads with three round green decorative attachments.

known as Trifari grew in reputation (continuing in business until modern times) and by 1930 was also producing large amounts of costume jewellery, sold through retail stores.

Many varieties of quartz were used in jewellery, the most precious being deep purple amethyst. Other types included yellow citrine, Scottish cairngorm and smoky quartz, the last of which can be confused with topaz, as well as rose quartz, rock crystal and rhinestones, which were originally rock crystal but were subsequently made of glass. In addition opals, jade and turquoise were much used, and there were jet imitations: these included French jet, which was black glass, vulcanite, a hard mouldable rubber, and Irish bog-oak.

Towards the end of the nineteenth century, following so much experimental production, what had previously given pleasure or shocked started to be regarded as boring, dull and of little appeal, sparking a frenetic search for novelty and renewed interest in jewellery. There was a revolt against mass-produced machine-made jewellery. Socialist ideals had become more acceptable and a desire had grown for simple, less expensive types of jewellery. The Art Nouveau influence was much to the fore from the 1880s and the distinctive styles of this phase, inspired by literature, art and natural forms, were extremely popular. Art Nouveau reached its peak at the Paris Exhibition in 1900, after which it rapidly lost popularity. Young women longed for the exotic in their increasing reaction against the rigidity and formality of the greater part of the nineteenth century. A turning point was the growth of the Arts and Crafts Movement, led by John Ruskin and his associate William Morris. They influenced designs in jewellery as well as in other fields, and this style continued to be fashionable into the twentieth century. Another major influence was the Glasgow School, especially Charles Rennie Mackintosh, and Liberty's of London, who were in the forefront of the avant-garde movement with their 'Cymric' designs.

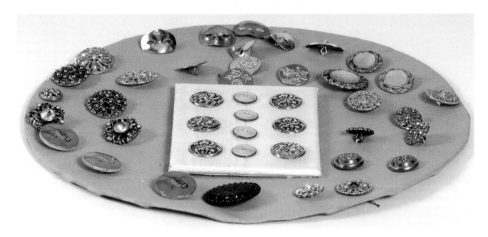

A collection of buttons. Across the top, in the centre, are five mask buttons – four of silver metal and one of brass. Below these are four engraved silver-on-metal two-piece buttons. To their right are one large and two smaller buttons with mother-of-pearl centres in cut-steel surrounds. To the far right are three matching cut-steel studded buttons. Along the bottom, the button in the centre is black French jet and to its left are three wooden buttons painted with blue tits. At the far top left are two flower-shaped cut-steel buttons, and in the centre, mounted on the fabric-covered card, is a set of six silver and four guilloche enamel buttons.

Buttons and buckles

Buttons have been used throughout most of history as a fastening for garments, but it was not until the nineteenth century that they came into their own as a complement to women's fashions and were to proliferate in an unprecedented manner. The demand in this period grew and the availability of new materials and new industrial processes made it possible to produce an infinite variety of more decorative buttons than had ever been seen before, to satisfy gentlemen and ladies who had money at their disposal.

For much of the period, cut steel was popular. Many designs were made in stamped-out metal, including the so-called 'mirror backs', in which the raised perforated top covers a reflective backing. Most buttons of this type were made in two pieces, a separate top fitted to a base with a looped shank for sewing on to a garment.

Enamel buttons were both beautiful and popular, as were those in hallmarked silver, many in Art Nouveau designs, often supplied in special boxes of matching sets. Mother-of-pearl buttons, large and small, some quite plain and others decoratively carved, were plentiful, as were glass buttons, among which buttons resembling paperweights – miniature versions of the items found on desks – are of especial interest. After the death of the Prince Consort, when the court was in mourning, large quantities of black fabric and glass buttons were

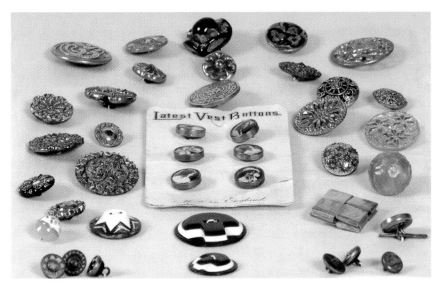

A varied collection of decorative buttons. The top two in the centre column are Bimini; the six to the left and right of the bottom row are Austrian Tinies. The six 'Latest Vest Buttons' on the card in the centre feature portraits of model women. Below these are two black and white plastic buttons from the late 1930s and, to their left, a purple and white plastic example from the same decade. Above the Austrian Tinies on the right is a square button made of cellophane paper, and, above to its right, a round one of similar composition. These date from the Second World War and just afterwards, when materials for button making were in very short supply. Among the remaining buttons are black, gold, coloured and white lustre glass; mirror backs; perforated pressed brass; cut steel; and an oval yellow glass example with white flower-decorated top.

A display of buttons. Across the top are five matching brass 'Paris backs', so called because they are marked 'Paris' on the back; these are flower-painted to resemble enamel. Below these, in the centre, are three champlevé enamel examples. Below again, in the middle of the centre column (from top), are a flower-decorated enamel, a flower-decorated porcelain and a Japanese Satsuma example. Below and to the left of the first Paris back is a cloisonné example. Along the bottom are three hallmarked silver Art Nouveau designs, plus a smaller similar one above the centre button. The remaining buttons incorporate plain or smoky mother-of-pearl in varied settings, and there are three set with paste stones.

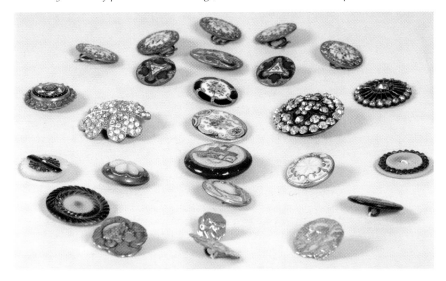

27

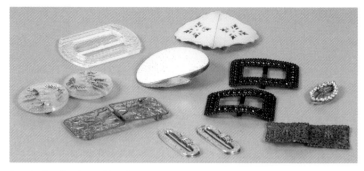

A mixed collection of buckles. (Clockwise from far left) Round painted glass; plain pressed glass; ostrich egg mounted on brass; hallmarked silver nurse's buckle, dated 1960, included to show an example; pair of rectangular French jet; small elliptical shape set with paste stones; lightweight link type, of elaborately decorated pressed metal; pair of nineteenth-century silver shoe buckles; pressed-brass link type.

made, some being relieved with lustre decoration. Lithograph buttons are another interesting type, these having a small subject or portrait print set in a metal mount under glass or clear celluloid, sometimes surrounded by facets in cut steel or by paste jewels. Small dress buttons in numerous varied designs were much used, one type being known as Austrian Tinies. There is a wide range of buttons made of painted or plain pressed-out metal, cut steel, ceramic, ivory, horn or wood and later of plastic, after various types of this material were developed. Buttons in tortoiseshell with piqué, hardstones and the distinctive Japanese Satsuma designs were also popular.

Buckles for shoes and belts were also made in variety, featuring many of the materials used for other items. One hallmarked silver type was given to young nurses when they achieved their State Registration, but there are also other silver examples, many in Art Nouveau designs. Cut steel was much used, as were, in later times, mother-of-pearl and plastics.

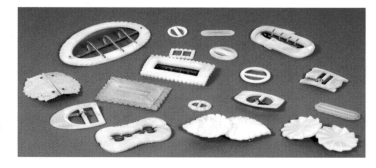

A collection of mother-of-pearl buckles, several with metal teeth to secure the belt and others with loops through which to thread the belt, to be secured with stitches.

Buttonhooks and shoehorns

The word 'buttonhook' is self-explanatory – a hook-shaped instrument to facilitate the pulling of buttons through buttonholes – but the reason for the widespread use of buttonhooks is less obvious. They were made in a variety of sizes, from a large, heavy type 10–12 inches (254–305 mm) long to one as short as 1¹/₂ to 3 inches (38–76 mm). During the nineteenth century the demands of fashion occasioned the increasing use of buttonhooks and their consequent mass production. In the late Victorian period and the early twentieth century women wore boots made of soft leather, which would cling to the ankle and show it off. These were fastened at the side with a number of buttons. Stiff corsets made bending difficult, so a buttonhook was a valuable accessory. Medium-sized hooks could be used for footwear but were also used, in the mid nineteenth century, to fasten the numerous buttons running from neck to hips on the bodices of dresses. The correct style of dress in the Victorian and Edwardian periods laid great emphasis on the type, colour and length of gloves to be worn, with certain styles accompanying particular outfits depending on the time of day. Many of the long gloves had as many as fifteen small buttons, and from 1835 onwards another type, with a small slit over the wrist, had four buttons to fasten. Thus the smallest hooks, used for this purpose, are known as glove hooks. These could be quite delicate – as their task was not so heavy as that of boot and shoe hooks – and could be made completely in silver or gold, but most have steel hooks embedded in small decorative handles. The larger buttonhooks also had steel hooks,

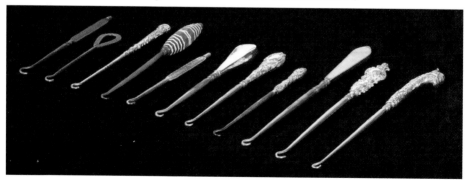

Boot and shoe buttonhooks. (Left to right) Iron, inscribed 'LE GRAND'S FRENCH DRESSING'; looped metal, inscribed 'MURPHY and BENNETT AND CO DECATUR, TEXAS'; silver with polished hook, marked steel; bronze hook, handle banded brown, cream and copper; steel, inscribed 'MANFIELDS BOOTS', with firm's name and address on reverse side; three silver, Birmingham, 1924, 1901 and 1921; pink enamel on silver, Birmingham, 1921; large silver, Birmingham, 1907; and another large silver, the hallmark very worn.

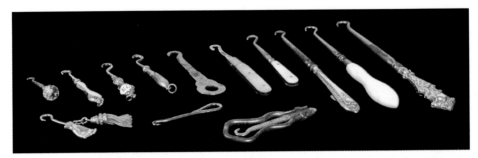

A collection of glove and dress buttonhooks. (Top row, left to right) Miniature brass glove hook with carved, round citrine top; two silver glove hooks, Birmingham, 1900; silver glove hook, Birmingham, 1906, with blue lace agate stone set in the handle; plain steel dress hook; silver hook folding into mother-of-pearl handle; steel hook with mother-of-pearl handle; silver dress hook, Sheffield, 1905; ivory; and silver. (Bottom row, left to right) Small novelty glove hook, hand-shaped with silver tassel; miniature polished steel; nickel-plated folding hook, the top of the hook shank marked 'MANDOLIN'.

some with steel handles, but many with handles of silver, silver plate, brass, ivory, mother-of-pearl, enamel, jet, bone, wood or semi-precious hardstones, such as coral, amethyst and banded agate. The handles of the hooks frequently feature novelties, such as birds (especially owls), fish, animals, boots or even Punch and Judy. Aside from its basic function of fastening buttons, the use of a buttonhook was also desirable in reducing the soiling of gloves by repeated use of the fingers.

With the growth of the travel industry in the late nineteenth century, buttonhooks became another souvenir item. Important events were frequently commemorated in the handles. Art Nouveau designs were often used in 1900–10, and the distinctive styles of Art Deco decoration were prevalent in the 1930s. The ingenuity in the design and shape of handles is endless. One less common type is a buttoner – instead of a hook, a variously shaped looped wire of a size to fit over a button was set in the handle, perhaps to be used for fastening spats (worn by ladies as well as gentlemen). A number of cheap base-metal hooks were used as small change or were made to be given away, advertising a particular product or shop.

Since the invention of the zip-fastener, long hooks could be used to fasten the back openings of dresses, being hooked into the tab of the zip; but the former, more general, use of the hooks died out with the change in fashion of dress, which largely did not need their help.

Buttonhooks can be found attached to shoehorns, a common instrument used to ease the foot into a boot or shoe. During the nineteenth century, although not so widely used as buttonhooks, shoehorns were especially useful because of the fashion for close-fitting footwear. Most shoehorns were originally made of horn,

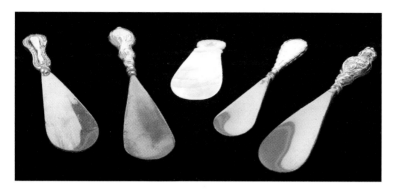

A group of shoehorns. (Left to right) Silver, Chester, 1917, horn marked English-made steel; Art Nouveau continental silver; rare, delicate mother-of-pearl; silver, 1911, and floral-decorated silver, 1938, both assayed in Birmingham.

but some were made in silver, brass, steel, ivory and even mother-of-pearl, many of these materials being used for decorating the handles. Horn is still used for the manufacture of shoehorns in the twenty-first century, particularly in Cumbria, though plastics are more often the material used. Shoehorns are kept in shoe shops for the use of customers trying on footwear. In the past they were often used to advertise well-known firms, for instance the shoe shops Manfield, Freeman Hardy & Willis and Trueform, as well as large department stores. They did not advertise only footwear-related products.

Some designs are small, and the horn, with or without a hook, is made to swivel into the handle so that it can be carried in a pocket and opened out for use. Another type was made to fold into a handle like a penknife (sometimes a blade was included), or into a pear-shaped handle.

Hatpins and hatpin holders

Hatpins are fashion accessories that became popular (and necessary) in the 1880s when Victorian bonnets were replaced by large flat hats placed on the top of the head. Anyone who has handled one of the long hatpins – up to 12 inches (305 mm) in length – which have become collectors' items, can readily

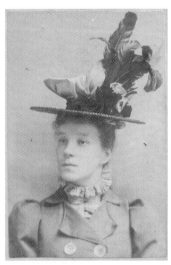

appreciate how dangerous they could be in crowded situations. Injuries were not infrequent, and the pins could be used as defensive weapons. By 1900 hats had become even larger, often featuring heavy decorations, and hairstyles too had changed to suit the new hats. Strong, fairly long pins were now necessary – 6–8 inches (152–203 mm) long – several being used for one hat, and around this time decorative tops to the pins started to appear. By 1911 the size of some hats had increased to 24 inches (610 mm) in diameter, requiring pins that were 16 inches (410 mm) long. By-laws were introduced to avoid injury to other people, and in 1913 notices appeared on public transport warning of the danger. Point protectors were produced, usually shaped like an acorn. By 1914 the pins had become smaller and in the 1920s they were reduced to 3 inches (76 mm), in keeping with the smaller styles of hat and bobbed hair then fashionable. Large hatpins finally

A lady in a jacket with leg-of-mutton sleeves, wearing a typical very large, flat hat, decorated with feathers, of the type secured by long hatpins, probably early twentieth century.

A boxed set of hatpins. Two long steel pins, the left-hand one with a smoky pearl top and the right-hand one being amber coloured. In the centre, the short pin on the right has a light blue top and the one on the left has a yellow top. The maker's name appears inside the silk-lined lid.

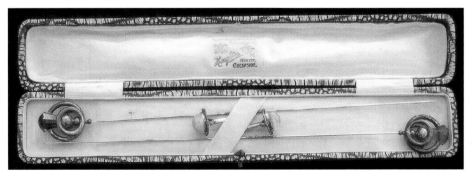

disappeared from use after the First World War when less formal styles of dress were worn.

Decorative hatpin tops vary in size from $^1/_2$ inch to $2^1/_2$ inches (13–63 mm) and were made in many different materials, such as porcelain (including Japanese Satsuma), gold, silver, tortoiseshell with piqué, mother-of-pearl, ivory, enamel, paste, semi-precious stones, cut steel, bone and Bakelite, after its introduction in 1907. The designs themselves are colourful, ingenious and of infinite variety. There were several special types, such as swivel or hinged tops, which could lie flat against the side of the hat.

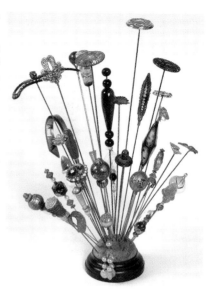

Right: A varied collection of long and short hatpins, the tops made of different materials, displayed in an ebony-based pincushion. Includes: malachite set in silver (back, third from left); a tall shaped Satsuma (to its right); RAF wings (far right, third from bottom); and a round flat-pressed French jet (back, to the right below the tallest pin).

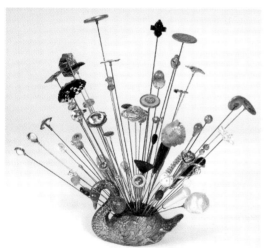

Below: A group of hatpins displayed in an Imari style pottery stand. Includes: a flower-shaped pair, silver with enamel; a Whitby jet horseshoe; a pair of Satsuma pins, featuring Japanese ladies; plain and bud-shaped mother-of-pearl.

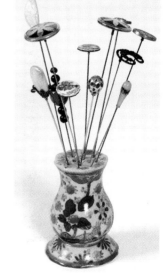

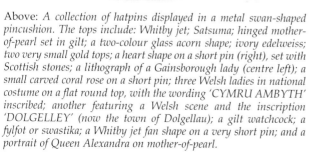

Above: A collection of hatpins displayed in a metal swan-shaped pincushion. The tops include: Whitby jet; Satsuma; hinged mother-of-pearl set in gilt; a two-colour glass acorn shape; ivory edelweiss; two very small gold tops; a heart shape on a short pin (right), set with Scottish stones; a lithograph of a Gainsborough lady (centre left); a small carved coral rose on a short pin; three Welsh ladies in national costume on a flat round top, with the wording 'CYMRU AMBYTH' inscribed; another featuring a Welsh scene and the inscription 'DOLGELLEY' (now the town of Dolgellau); a gilt watchcock; a fylfot or swastika; a Whitby jet fan shape on a very short pin; and a portrait of Queen Alexandra on mother-of-pearl.

Animal shapes, birds, butterflies, fruit, flowers and buildings can all be found, together with button tops, both decorative and regimental, the latter appearing during the First World War. In 1902 teddy-bear tops started to appear following an incident on a shooting expedition, when President Theodore Roosevelt refused to shoot a bear cub, which subsequently became known as 'Teddy'. After 1905 tops were made with semi-precious stones and had silver bands, insect motifs and sporting designs, such as ice-skates and roller-skates, tennis rackets, hockey sticks, golf clubs and hunting emblems; the sporting models became popular as women had started to take part in sports when the rigid Victorian way of life had begun to be cast aside. In 1911 hatpin tops appeared with the fylfot or tetraskelion motif (most familiar as the swastika), which is a symbol of good fortune. With the gradual increase of travel possibilities people brought back all kinds of souvenirs from their holidays, and hatpins were no exception. Souvenir hatpins featured Cornish serpentine, jet from Whitby in Yorkshire, bog-oak and Connemara marble from Ireland, and semi-precious stones from Scotland. Souvenir tops were also made, featuring the coats of arms of cities, photographs of cathedrals, maps, the three-legged symbol of the Isle of Man, the Lincoln imp, the shamrock emblem of Ireland, the Union Jack, Australian kangaroos and enamelled Canadian maple-leaves, to name but a few examples. There were a number of specialist makers, with their own individual designs.

Among the most sought-after hatpins are those with hallmarked silver tops made by Charles Horner of Halifax, a most prolific producer, often in Art Nouveau designs. Some using enamel were particularly characteristic of the late nineteenth century. The hallmark consists of the mark for the Chester assay office and the initials 'CH' for Charles Horner, followed by a date letter.

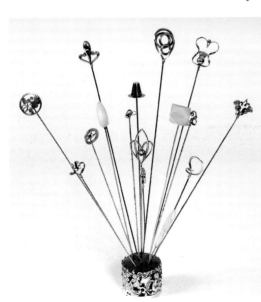

The steel or nickel-plated shafts of the pins vary in shape, some having a plain pointed end, some a flat bayonet-shaped point and others a spiral shaft.

A small group of hatpins displayed in a silver pincushion, Birmingham, 1901; these are silver, some hallmarked, and two have mother-of-pearl tops. The round one (far left) has a green enamel trefoil with blue leaves; below it, to the right, is a round mauve enamel buckle made by Charles Horner, 1912, hinged to lie flat against the hat. Other pins of note are the Welsh hat (centre); and the long one with the brown glass thistle (top right), Birmingham, 1909.

34

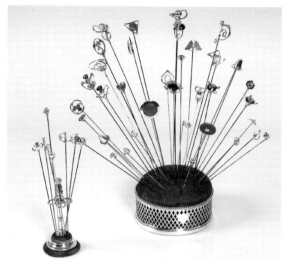

Two collections of silver hatpins, assayed in Chester and made by Charles Horner, a much sought-after type; a number of distinctive Art Nouveau designs, displayed in a small silver hatpin stand, Birmingham, 1908 (left), and a large red silver-based pincushion (right). Some tops are enamel on silver; some have semi-precious stones, amethyst, citrine, coral and malachite. There are two Welsh-hat-shaped tops, a butterfly, several thistle tops and a halberd. The smaller pins, low down in front, have gold tops. Most of the pins are very long steel ones of the early years of the twentieth century.

The tops were attached according to what they were made of; for example, porcelain tops had the shaft glued in, silver tops had a type of hollow collar to secure the top, and tortoiseshell or other natural materials were riveted on to a silver collar.

The most effective way to display a collection of hatpins is in a large weighted pincushion, but a great variety of stands and holders was made to store personal pins and can now be used for display. Some hatpin holders were made in silver, silver plate or brass, often in novelty designs, but they usually consist of a central rod fitted with a number of rings, attached to a base plate fitted with a velvet-covered pincushion or a wire mesh. The pins could be placed through the rings and secured in the cushion or mesh. The tops of the central rods were decorated in various ways. There are many china hatpin holders; these were usually vase-shaped with a large central hole surrounded by smaller holes. There are many types of decoration, including crested china souvenir designs.

A group of hatpin holders. (Left to right) Metal shoe pincushion with roundel featuring 'LOWESTOFT' below the laces; white china made in Czechoslovakia, with forget-me-not decoration; Imari-style pottery; silver stand, Birmingham, 1908; and typical Devon pottery with the message 'I'll take care of the pins'.

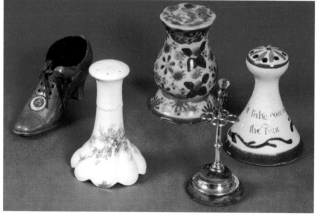

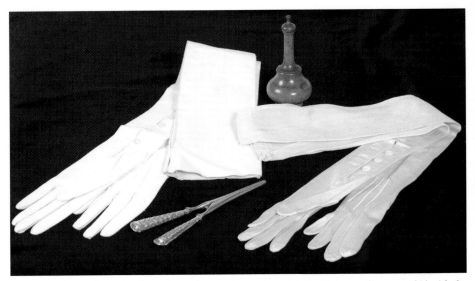

Two pairs of long above-the-elbow gloves, buttoned over the wrist. (Left) A very fine cream kid with the typical four buttons. (Right) An unworn pair in very fine knitted cream silk, with three buttons and the original price tag of 6s 11d (approximately 35p). With these is a boxwood glove-powdering flask, which would have been valuable after kid gloves had been washed, with its original screw-on cap, and a pair of silver-handled glove stretchers, Birmingham, 1911, with the registered number 580393; these would also have been invaluable for kid gloves.

Gloves, glove stretchers, powdering flasks and glove boxes

Throughout the nineteenth and early twentieth centuries gloves were an important dress accessory, being worn for daytime or evening in varying lengths. White kid was popular, and special boxes were used to keep them clean and neat. Some were simply a wooden or papier-mâché box, painted or fabric-covered, but a more interesting type, usually covered in leather but occasionally silk, was expanding, with concertina sides. Some have a fitted space inside the lid to hold glove stretchers and sometimes a buttonhook.

Glove stretchers were used to restore the shape of glove fingers after washing, which made them wrinkled and stiff. The stretchers were made in boxwood, rosewood and ebony, but also ivory, tortoiseshell, bone and brass. There are wooden examples in Scottish Tartan and Mauchline souvenir wares. The Tartan type are decorated with Tartan patterned paper and the Mauchline ones are made in pale sycamore wood with a black transfer print of some resort or place of interest. The earliest type of glove stretcher had no spring between the handles, but later ones had this improvement. Another fairly common variety was

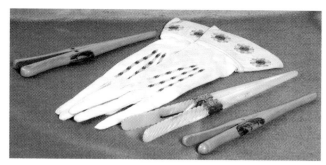

Three pairs of glove stretchers with a pair of fine cream kid gloves with flower-embroidered gauntlet and backs. (Left to right) Mauchline, sycamore wood with a black transfer print, 'Panorama or Double View, Barmouth'; fine quality mother-of-pearl with silver banding; another Mauchline pair, with the transfer print 'Jedburgh Abbey'.

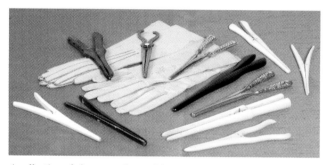

A collection of glove stretchers with two pairs of fine glacé kid gloves, the lower pair embroidered on the backs. (Clockwise from top left) Tortoiseshell; engraved brass with decorative white centre button; silver, Birmingham, 1911, with leaf decoration; ebony; silver, Birmingham, 1906; two ivory pairs. (Top right) Ivory; very small slim bone. (Bottom) Ivory (far left) and (next to it) wood.

made in steel with silver or ivory handles. Some glove stretchers will be found in boxed sets with a matching shoe horn.

The long gloves could be quite difficult to put on, and to simplify this it was usual to powder the insides, and for this a special glove-powdering flask was made of boxwood, ebony or ivory. The flasks were shaped like a small bulbous bottle, the neck being screwed into the top of the bulb shape, which held the powder. The top of the long neck part was pierced with holes like a pepper pot, and some can be found with the screw-on cap for this, though frequently these have been lost.

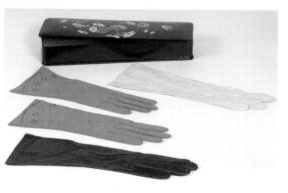

A papier-mâché glove box, the lid painted with a blue tit and daisies. Below it are four travellers' sample kid gloves – cream, two tan and brown – the labels giving sizes.

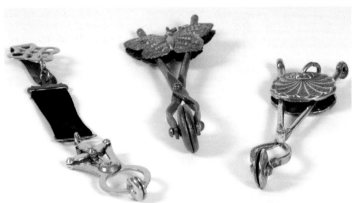

Three skirt lifters. (Left to right) A patent spring type, marked 'DEPOSÉ', with chatelaine hook and black silk moiré ribbon; brass, with a central butterfly motif, the circular grips marked 'Registered Sept. 1876'; brass, with a central shell motif, the discs ornamentally engraved.

Skirt lifters

Means of managing long skirts to prevent soiling had been known for a long time, but it was during the nineteenth century that the gadgets known as 'skirt lifters' or 'pages' became popular; thousands were produced to deal not only with long skirts but also with the very full ones that were then fashionable.

During the nineteenth century, road drainage was haphazard (macadam surfacing had not yet been introduced), and uncollected garbage was thrown out into the unswept streets, so that fashionable skirts, often made of costly and delicate materials, could be easily soiled. Furthermore, methods for washing or dry-cleaning garments that we now take for granted were not then available. In addition, dresses had to last and therefore needed care. Some ladies were able to drive in a carriage or chaise or might use the services of a crossing sweeper, who had to be given a tip. Safety pins were patented in 1876, but a more efficient means of assistance was necessary and in the last quarter of the century skirt lifters were invented; these were useful for avoiding damage to delicate fabrics by continual hoisting up from the ground by the hands. They were ingenious devices, looking rather like a pair of strange scissors: two pivoted arms ending in cushioned circles, which could be locked by a contrivance at the top between the two arms and operated by a cord suspended from the waist. A corner of the skirt hem was placed between the discs, which were then locked tight, and a pull on the cord lifted the skirt free of the ground. A number of different types existed and the locking devices were decorated in a variety of ways; hands, butterflies, horseshoes, hearts and peacocks are just a few of the many designs popular. Skirt lifters were mainly made in non-precious metals, usually brass or plated. Some models had a miniature version attached and there were a number of different makes, one well-known example being Fyfes Patent.

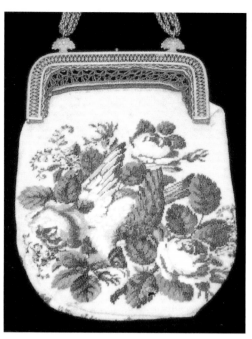

A fine-quality beaded purse on an elaborate gold frame, with part-beaded openwork and a double gold-chain handle. The design is of a bird with leaves and flowers.

Handbags, purses and chatelaines

Most late-twentieth-century women would have felt lost without a handbag, that valuable accessory in which a woman carried all the paraphernalia seemingly indispensable to her daily life, although towards the end of that century many young women had to a large extent dispensed with them.

It was not until 1880 that the first leather handbags were made and became popular. Earlier in the nineteenth century fashions in clothes had dictated the means of carrying the items necessary for the comfort and convenience of a lady. When skirts were full they often concealed pockets made as part of the dress or tied on separately, but when skirts were slim and clinging some other form had to be used, as pockets would have caused unsightly and uncomfortable bulges.

By 1850 the age of rail travel had begun. This was not very comfortable at first, so bags were useful for carrying necessities. In addition, the crinolines of the 1850s and 1860s meant there was a need for more bags, some of which were fabric chatelaine types that could be hung from a hook at the waist or carried by a finger ring; these continued in use until the 1890s. The bags were mainly square and flat and one use was to carry a visiting-card case. Beaded purses had been popular, but around 1860 and throughout the Victorian period 'long purses' were widely used. These purses were of a slim sausage shape, early ones netted and

39

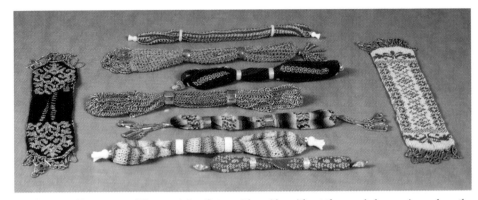

A collection of long purses. The ones lying flat on either side, without the usual closure rings, show the elaborate beaded patterns and fringing. In the centre row (top to bottom), the second, third, fourth and last all have coloured, steel or gilt beads and steel or gilt closure rings. These purses have an open slit in the centre through which to enclose coins, with a ring slid down and then moved up to hold the coins safely. The purse at the top is two-colour crochet with unusual mother-of-pearl closure rings and finials; and the second from the bottom is also crochet, with unusual ivory closure rings. The green, red and yellow one third from bottom is of very fine knitted material.

later ones crocheted in silk, decorated with beads and often with bead tassels; green was the most popular colour. Two rings could be slid along to hold the coins in each end away from the central opening. Very tiny round purses in brass, mother-of-pearl or tortoiseshell, some made to hang from a hand-held chain or from one attached to a chatelaine hook, were made to carry a few small coins, of the small size of the period.

The chatelaine had a revival in the 1870s when narrow skirts were fashionable. Chatelaines were made in a variety of materials, mainly silver, silver plate, brass or steel, with a few less common types such as leather. They consisted of a large central pierced or engraved motif with a hook to attach to the waistband, from which were suspended a number of chains, usually three, five, or sometimes seven, to which could be attached useful small accessories, such as a scent bottle, pencil, penknife, tweezers or notebook. The later ones mostly carried needlework items: a thimble in a case, a needle-case, a pincushion, and scissors in a sheath. A choice of accessories could be bought to attach to the rings or swivel clips on the end of the chains; there was a well-known shop in Bond Street, London, that sold the necessary items. Chatelaines continued to be worn until the end of the nineteenth century, including the period when full-skirted dresses with a normal waistline were in fashion, but they gradually became heavier and less attractive in design. A number may have been worn more for effect than necessity: they were expensive so it was mainly well-off women who wore them. The Victorian housewife liked to imagine herself as the mistress of the house or castle, like the original medieval 'chatelaine' – the lady of the castle – for whom this item

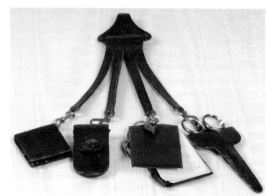

An unusual black leather chatelaine in mint condition, with four items on leather hanging straps. (Left to right) pincushion; needle-packet holder with press-stud closure; notebook; scissors in a sheath.

Right: *Two silver chatelaines. (Left) Birmingham, 1897, with three decorative chains ending in swivel clips, holding (left to right): small glove buttonhook with blue lace agate stone in the handle, 1906; heart-shaped pincushion, 1900; aide-mémoire in silver covers, 1911. All assayed in Birmingham. (Right) Hallmarked Birmingham, 1901, with four plain chains with swivel clips, containing (left to right): silver penknife, Birmingham, 1911; scent bottle in a silver holder, Chester, 1898; small glove buttonhook, Birmingham, 1900; silver pencil with amethyst stone in the top.*

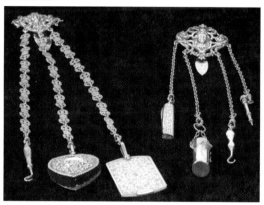

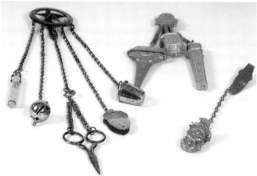

Left: *Two chatelaines and a skirt lifter. (Left) Steel, dating from the mid nineteenth century, with five chains ending in split rings, holding (left to right): needle-case; spherical tape-measure; scissors; acorn-shaped pincushion; thimble in thimble bucket. (Centre) An elaborate pinchbeck chatelaine, carrying three items (left to right): scissors in lidded sheath; lidded thimble bucket with original matching thimble; lidded needle-case. This chatelaine has a dedication inscription on the back dated 8th June 1892. (Right) A metal chatelaine-type skirt lifter.*

was an essential piece of equipment. Suspended from the chatelaine's waist would have been a hook with chains on which she carried the keys to the wooden chests, which stored precious, expensive tea and sugar, to prevent theft by her servants, cupboards not then having been introduced. In time the name passed from the wearer herself to the actual object.

In 1890 the term 'handbag' was first used for a bag that was carried rather than worn. Prior to that it had only been used to

41

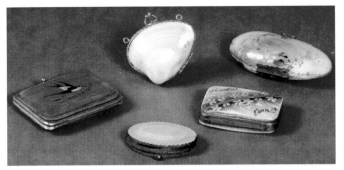

Three souvenir and two mother-of-pearl purses. (Clockwise from left) Wooden, with 'Nice' on the back and a swallow in flight above the word 'Souvenir' on the front, with twist-knob closure; natural shell with gilt-metal mounts, twist-knob closure and loops for a carrying chain, missing; bivalve shell purse painted with flowers (worn), with brass hinge and fastening, metal mounts and carrying chain, the interior partitions and lining made of red paper simulated leather; mother-of-pearl, painted with 'A present from' above a diagonal strip of blue and white flowers and then 'Conway', with twist-knob fastening, silver-metal mounts and red paper lining and partitions; leather purse with carved mother-of-pearl ovals on the back and front.

A collection of metal purses. (Clockwise from bottom left) Steel chain; heavier, darker, similar example; bright metal; oval with brass frame, miniature cut-steel beads and twist-knob fastener; small gilt-metal chain. (Centre) Engraved brass frame, with small brass studs stitched together, lined in brown suede, and with a twist-knob fastening.

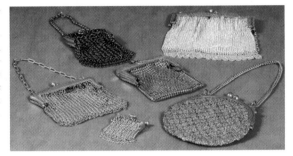

distinguish it from leather luggage. From then on bags began to resemble those recognised in modern times. Between 1890 and 1900 bags of steel mesh on a metal frame were popular. By the end of the nineteenth century the use of face powder was just becoming acceptable and powder compacts began to appear. These and the double-ended scent bottle, with perfume in one end and restorative salts in the other, were a boon in hot and crowded ballrooms and theatres, so decorative bags were needed to carry the items, perhaps along with dainty opera glasses.

During the First World War and around 1919, Dorothy bags were popular. These were mainly made of fabrics or soft leather, with a drawstring to close them; others had frames of tortoiseshell, which had been substituted for the metal needed for the war effort. After the war women rapidly became more independent. Many had for the first time been employed in wartime work, and many changes were taking place. Women began to wear make-up in public – lipstick, rouge and eye make-up – and smoking became acceptable, so the types of bag carried reflected the need for the associated items. By 1914 the first metal

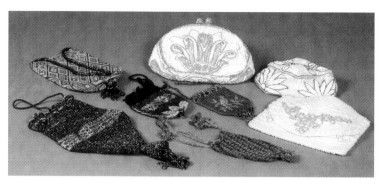

A collection of beaded purses. (Clockwise from top left) Large, with small multicoloured beads in diamond pattern with beaded handle and bottom tassel; gold and white beads, twist-knob fastening; flower design with flap, the petals made from pearlised white beads edged with black bugle beads, on a background of mother-of-pearl bugles, with a wrist loop at the back; pale blue and white beads mounted on silk, made by the owner; small dark blue and gold netted drawstring purse, the drawstring and the bottom of the purse finished with flowers in gold thread; large, mainly blue-beaded, with a corded drawstring to close. (Centre) Small flower-decorated blue with black crochet top and drawstring (left); bronze and green with green cord drawstring and looped green fringe at the bottom (right).

Four purses made in complex-design petit point embroidery, one with a 'loom made' label inside, on decorative gilt frames with twist-knob closures and carrying cords. The fifth purse (bottom left) is crocheted in blue and white thread and has a tortoiseshell frame, a snap closure and a carrying cord.

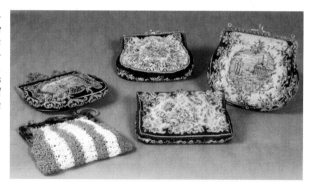

clasps had appeared, followed in 1919 by the first, rather heavy, zip-fasteners, which did gradually reduce in weight. By 1920 the zip was regarded as being necessary for security.

After the 1920s plastics were introduced, including casein (a milk product) and Xylonite (an ivory substitute), and these were used in the making of bags. The bag was by now an integral part of a woman's outfit, and in the middle of the period the pochette appeared on the scene, replacing medium-sized handbags. This was a flat, medium-sized purse with a flap front, and was carried under the arm or in the hand. A vertical loop was soon attached to the back of the purse to slip over the wrist for additional security. The pochette continued to be popular until 1936.

Over the years many changes in the design, shape, size and materials of the handbag have occurred and during the Second World War the first shoulder bags with long handles made their appearance.

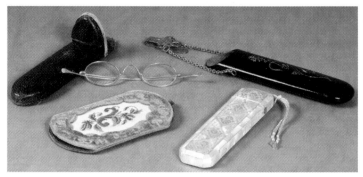

Four spectacle cases with a pair of early oval gold-rimmed spectacles. (Clockwise from bottom left) Double slip-in case, the inner section made of simulated leather-covered card with a pull tab, fitting into an outer case of velvet fabric with impressed decoration, covering a rose-embroidered inset on the front and a pansy on the back; frog-mouth case, covered with simulated leather, belonging to the spectacles below it; papier-mâché case with painted decoration and chatelaine clip; fine mother-of-pearl case with hinged top and carrying cord.

Spectacles, quizzing glasses and lorgnettes

Bygone spectacles were mostly somewhat different in style to the modern versions, usually having flattened oval-shaped lenses, K- or X-shaped bridge styles, either with or without side-pieces, and occasionally folding. They could be slipped into slim cases of a suitable shape.

In the middle of the nineteenth century spectacles were made of steel wire, which was treated with heat to prevent rusting. Although reasonably priced spectacles had become available,

Folding lorgnettes and quizzing glasses. (Top from left) Gold glass with round lens and reef-knot handle; folding lorgnette with smoky pearl handle and chain; 9 carat gold chased frame glass with oval lens; silver folding lorgnette with ring to attach to ribbon or chain. (Bottom from left) Gold-framed rectangular-shaped glass with figure-of-eight handle; continental silver folding lorgnette; 9 carat gold folding lorgnette with elegant trefoil-decorated handle.

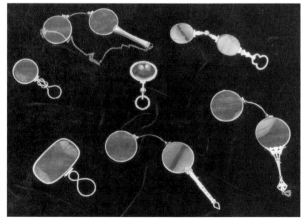

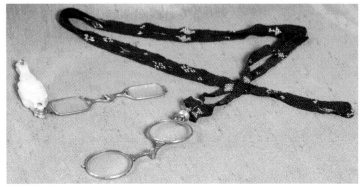

Fine mother-of-pearl folding lorgnette with rectangular lenses (left), and round-lensed brass-rimmed spectacles on a long black and gold beaded cord (right).

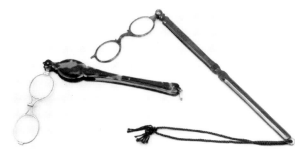

Left: *Lorgnettes. (Left) Folding tortoiseshell-handled example, held closed with a metal fastener. (Right) Rigid eyepieces that fold straight down into an imitation-tortoiseshell handle.*

ladies of this time were ashamed of needing them and did not like to be seen in them, preferring instead to use quizzing glasses, which could show off graceful movement. The early ones had small round lenses set in gold with a short handle; later more ornate ones, oval or oblong in shape, became popular, being worn on a ribbon or a cord. Lorgnettes also were desirable, the early ones being made of gold, tortoiseshell, ivory or mother-of-pearl, and having a short handle into which the lenses folded. At the end of the 1870s styles with longer handles, which lent themselves to display, were much used; these were sometimes straight and flat, and sometimes folding, and were again made in gold, silver, pinchbeck, mother-of-pearl or tortoiseshell, with or without piqué decoration. In 1875 pince-nez were widely worn, but by the end of the nineteenth century rimless spectacles were the most popular type, being relatively inconspicuous. In 1935 a dress-clip lorgnette was developed, which could be clipped on to a garment and easily opened in order to read menus or programmes.

Card cases, aides-mémoire and notebooks

Card cases were used throughout the nineteenth century and into the twentieth, but the majority to be found date from 1850 onwards, when production was at its height. Members of upper- and middle-class society spent the 'season' in London and the remainder of the year at their homes out of town, visiting or entertaining. Calling and leaving a card was an important, carefully regulated and prescribed activity, occupying much of the time of leisured ladies, who had servants to deal with the running of their homes. It was considered essential to make one's way in society, and for families there was the overriding consideration of marrying their sons and daughters in the right spheres. To be successful in this aim meant following the correct codes of behaviour and being known in the right company. Books on etiquette for the period give precise instructions for all occasions, and on all aspects of calling and leaving cards. The cards had to be of a specified size for ladies and gentlemen, those for ladies being the larger. They had to be printed in a carefully prescribed way, and for mourning they were required to be edged with a black band of regulation width.

Card cases were made in a wide variety of materials, including hallmarked silver, mother-of-pearl – some incorporating abalone shell in a pattern of diamond-shaped panes – and tortoiseshell, both these last two often having silver inlays, and the tortoiseshell having silver or gold piqué. Cameo carving or fretted designs in mother-of-pearl were also frequently used, as were plain or carved ivory, papier-mâché, lacquer decorated with mother-of-pearl inlay, painted wood, and souvenir Tunbridge, Tartan or Mauchline ware. Other materials used include deeply carved sandalwood, which could have inlays of shell, steel or ivory; marquetry; Bois Durci (a composition made to look like wood); leather-covered

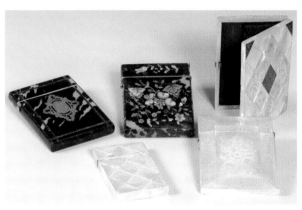

A group of ladies' card cases. (Clockwise from top left) Tortoiseshell with hinged lid and silver cartouche for initials; tortoiseshell with hinged lid, decorated with inlaid mother-of-pearl flowers and leaves; open, a case decorated with engraved diamond-shaped mother-of-pearl panels with silver cartouche and corners, hinged at the back with a snap fastening, lined with royal blue silk and having gilt-edged royal blue partitions; a very fine-quality mother-of-pearl case with decoration of high relief carving and a hinged lid; mother-of-pearl with diamond-shaped panels and hinged lid.

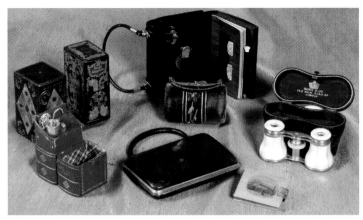

A varied group of useful cases. (Clockwise from bottom left) Open Lady's Companion, covered in red leatherette, containing sewing items – needle-case, scissors, stiletto, thimble – also a pencil, a knife and, on the right, a red velvet-covered pincushion; two other Lady's Companions, the second with gold lettering and containing an incomplete set of sewing items, and the first with a complete set inside as previously described plus matching tweezers and buttonhook slotted into one side of the needle-case, as well as a simulated ivory and tortoiseshell memorandum card with the name and address of the supplier in gilt lettering and a calendar for 1889 advertising wine and spirit merchants; a fine small handbag-style nécessaire containing a thimble, a purse with several compartments, a notebook and pencil, slots for stamps, a mirror with an ivory memo card slotted over it, scissors, looped buttoner, nail tools and ear spoon, needle-case, cards of coloured thread, and a flannel strip for needles and pins; Victorian mother-of-pearl and gilt-metal opera glasses with their original case; Mauchline notebook with black transfer print of the breakwater and entrance to the harbour, Watchet; handbag-style nécessaire made of leather on a metal frame. (Centre) Carrying-purse style nécessaire in purple velvet on a brass frame, with a silk pocket in one half and matching thimble, scissors and needle-case, and with a pencil and bodkins in a fitted partition in the other half.

card; straw work; and some early synthetics such as Bakelite. A number of these types were imported and they remind us that during the Victorian period the British Empire was expanding. Britons living abroad carried on their normal activities and so would use card cases made in local styles and materials. The spread of tourism made souvenir styles popular.

Aides-mémoire and notebooks are also collectable accessories, some having ivory and others paper leaves. They were made in many sizes and materials, some having a pencil slipped through loops at the side in order to enclose the leaves in covers of elaborately decorated silver, silver plate, mother-of-pearl or ivory. Sometimes the leaves are printed with the days of the

An engraved brass toothpick case lined with green velvet and a mother-of-pearl toothpick folding into a protective handle.

week; or those having 'Carnet de Bal' inscribed on the cover were dance pro-grammes in which to write the names of one's partners for individual dances.

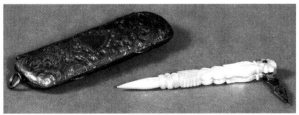

Posy holders

These attractive Victorian accessories have become extremely scarce and expensive. They were usually funnel-shaped and made in elaborately cut gold, silver or pinchbeck (a cheap substitute for gold made from zinc and copper and named after Christopher Pinchbeck, who invented it in the early eighteenth century). Sometimes they had mother-of-pearl handles, and a complete specimen should have a pin to secure the posy of fresh flowers and a ring or loop on a chain to be hung around the finger when dancing (or sometimes they were carried in the hand). Posies were not simply carried to be attractive, but also to counteract in hot and crowded ballrooms or other social gatherings the effects of poor standards of personal hygiene and the inevitably difficult cleaning of garments.

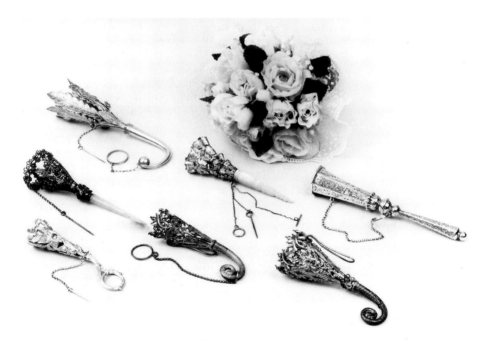

Posy holders, displayed with a typical posy. (Top row slanting from left to right) Continental silver, leaves forming a funnel that can be opened out wider or closed as shown, complete with pin to secure the posy and a finger ring; elaborate gilt metal in a frilled design with a mother-of-pearl handle, ring and pins; a very fine engraved continental silver example. (Centre row) Floral gilt-metal design with carved mother-of-pearl handle and pin; smaller gilt metal with curved handle and ring; another in gilt metal, probably pinchbeck, with curved handle and a hook by which the holder could be fastened over the belt. (Bottom left) Small continental silver type with pin and integral finger ring as the handle.

Fans

The earliest use of the fan was simply as a cooling aid, but as civilisation developed it came to have a much more complex ritual significance, especially in the Far East. As well as being useful, the fan ultimately acquired social importance, and the highest forms of art and craftsmanship were employed in making such a highly esteemed accessory. The leisured upper and middle classes indulged in frequent social activities. At dances and balls the atmosphere in crowded rooms could be hot and stuffy, which, in addition to the discomfort of constricting and uncomfortable clothing, must have made a fan a comfort indeed. It was, however, also a social attribute, requiring graceful movement of the hands and being capable of artful and eloquent use to convey emotions. In an age when the young of opposite sexes were not allowed to meet alone, words and glances could be exchanged under its cover, and a complete language of the fan was developed. To touch the fan with the tip of a finger meant 'I wish to speak to you'. Fans became increasingly fashionable in an era when it was socially acceptable to be affected, and if a lady was attending a play with some risqué content she could make good use of a type of fan called the 'lorgnette'. This had small holes in some of the guards, covered with glass or net, through which she could observe all that was going on, while apparently shielding her eyes.

There are two main types of fan: rigid and folding. The first had a single, shaped piece of material attached to a central stick. The material might be wood or papier-mâché with mother-of-pearl or painted decoration, or feathers or fabric decorated with painting or embroidery. This type was popular from 1840 onwards. Folding fans are made up of two outer guards and, in between, a number of sticks opening out into a semicircle, all held together by a pinion, to which may be attached a finger ring. This type is fitted with a single leaf of fabric, lace, very fine skin or paper decorated in a variety of ways, painted, embroidered or covered with sequins. One type of folding fan is called the 'brisé': this has small pieces of ribbon, inserted through slots in the sticks, and guards to link them

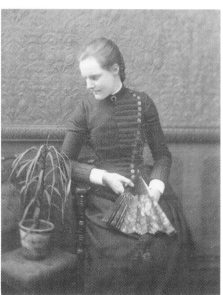

A lady in late Victorian black dress holding a fan.

49

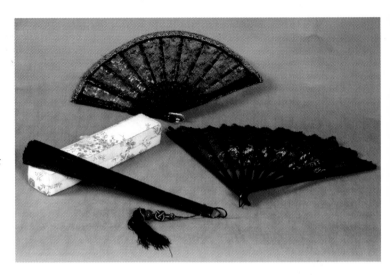

Three black fans with a fabric-covered box. The folded one on the box is black lace with a tassel; the open one at the back has gilt decoration on black gauze; and the one on the right is fine black lace with a floral decoration.

together. Another type is the 'cockade', which unfolds from inside the double handle and is adjusted by means of a slim cord. France was the chief centre for the manufacture of fans, although there were English makers. The name of Duvelleroy became famous in Britain after the Great Exhibition of 1851.

The rapid changes in styles of dress throughout the nineteenth century influenced the corresponding changes in the design and decoration of fans, which increased and decreased in size to match the size of skirts, and which changed in colour to reflect those most popular at a given time. Many fans were modelled on earlier styles; there were thicker sticks, lavishly gilded and decorated, and the types of heavier fabrics used for clothes as the century progressed were adapted for fans. In earlier times fans had been hand-painted, but printing was used later, and much in evidence also were Japanese and Chinese influences, for fans had great ceremonial significance in both Japan and China.

Around the middle of the nineteenth century fans were of small to medium size, 6–8 inches (150–200 mm), those for use out of doors often being small painted ones or sandalwood ones of the brisé type. Pierced ivory and wood for brisé fans were imported from China throughout the century. In the 1860s the sticks were rather wide, made of ivory, bone, wood or tortoiseshell, the leaf being decorated with spangles of steel cut in star or flower shapes. Leaves of bobbin and needle lace were also used at this time and continued to be popular until the end of the nineteenth century. Widely used in the late 1870s were broad heavy sticks in various shapes, with a leaf of silk or satin, trimmed, embroidered or painted. Feather fans, using cock, pigeon or pheasant plumage, were also popular. Another variety used was the folding circular 'parasol' fan. In the 1880s, very

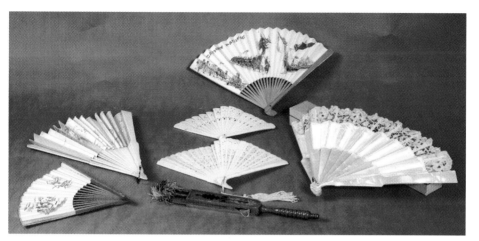

A collection of fans. (Clockwise from bottom left) Modern souvenir paper type on cedarwood sticks, with pictures of Spanish scenes, including dancing, bullfighting, horseback-riding and a Moorish town quarter, marked 'Cruises, Peninsula and Oriental Steam Navigation Company, Souvenir Ceuta, 1955'; ivory sticks with painted satin leaf; another souvenir paper type on cedarwood, with 'CATHAY PACIFIC' and pictures of the East; fine mother-of-pearl sticks with satin and lace leaf, resting on a card fan box. (Centre, top to bottom) Cream plastic brisé; ivory brisé with silk tassel; closed painted-wood cockade example.

large fans, some with smaller sticks at the sides, were fashionable. The 'ostrich feather' style was also used towards the end of the century, continuing into the early twentieth century, when popularity then turned towards smaller designs. In the 1880s and 1890s Honiton lace motifs appliquéd on to fine net were introduced, as was ready-made tape lace mounted on net, linked by stitches made with a needle.

The nineteenth-century styles of fans were gradually abandoned when fine-art decoration was superseded by Arts and Crafts styles in design and manufacture. Very few fans were painted during the Art Nouveau and Art Deco periods; the typical Art Nouveau patterns and colours were few and far between following the introduction of many cheap types on the market, and the formerly popular lace and feather fans began to disappear after the First World War as behaviour and styles of dress changed. There was less frivolity, and fans were made simply to amuse or for use in advertising. With the age of easier travel souvenir fans did appear, but the long period when the use of fans was fashionable gradually came to an end.

51

Parasols

Although parasols had been known throughout history, it was during the nineteenth century, when ladies became particularly concerned to preserve a delicate complexion in accordance with the attitudes of society, that this accessory enjoyed much more widespread popularity, being frequently seen when ladies were out walking or driving in carriages in bright sunshine. Another potential use, however, as an aid to flirtation, was appreciated by fashionable women.

The early parasols were small and dainty, covered in delicate fabrics such as silk or lace and often trimmed with silk fringes. The sticks were long and were finished with small handles made of ivory, mother-of-pearl or wood. One popular shape in the 1860s was the 'pagoda', and a special 'carriage' parasol was popular between 1837 and 1865. The handle was in two parts, hinged in the centre, and had a deep ring that could be slid up to secure the two parts.

As fashions changed in the second half of the nineteenth century, the small styles were superseded by larger types, covered in slightly heavier materials and more elaborately trimmed, with larger, heavier and thicker handles made of china, crystal or wood. These were often covered to match an outfit. Later still, they increased further in size and became more sturdy, with long handles, and were covered in materials that were even heavier, less elaborate in trim, and more gaudy in colour. This style continued until the late 1870s and 1880s, when the parasol grew longer and slimmer when closed and could be used as an umbrella.

Two folding carriage parasols. (Left) Black and gold silk with matching fringe, the wooden handle showing the folding mechanism. (Right) Cream embroidered silk cover lined with cream silk and with silk fringe, the wooden handle fully extended.

Parasols were still to be seen in the early part of the twentieth century. In 1901 the fashion was for sunshades with long handles topped by Art Nouveau style knobs, enamelled or featuring fruit, and covered in Chantilly lace, flowered or moiré silk. In 1921 sunshades of a flat, Japanese shape were to be seen, while in 1923 dumpy umbrellas to match the dress were in fashion. In 1939 organdie-covered lacy parasols were popular, again to match the dress, but after this the more utilitarian, if often quite elegant, style of umbrella superseded the formerly popular lighter types.

Further reading

Alexander, Hélène. *Fans*. Shire, second edition 2002.
Armstrong, Nancy. *A Collector's History of Fans*. Studio Vista, 1974.
Baker, Lillian. *Hatpins and Hatpin Holders*. Collector Books (Kentucky, USA), 1983.
Becker, Vivienne. *Antique and Twentieth Century Jewellery*. NAG Press, 1987.
Betensley, Bertha. *Antique Buttonhooks for Shoes, Gloves and Clothing*. Educator Press (USA), 1955; reprinted by Buttonhook Society, 1991.
Brandon, Sue. *Buttonhooks and Shoehorns*. Shire, 1984; reprinted 2000.
Buck, A. *Victorian Costume and Costume Accessories*. Herbert Jenkins, 1961.
Cunnington, C. Willett. *English Women's Clothing in the Present Century*. Faber & Faber, 1952.
Davidson, D. C., and MacGregor, R. J. S. *Spectacles, Lorgnettes and Monocles*. Shire, second edition 2002.
Foster, Vanda. *Bags and Purses*. Batsford, The Costume Accessories Series, 1982.
Hinks, Peter. *Nineteenth Century Jewellery*. Faber & Faber, 1975.
Houart, Victor. *Buttons: A Collector's Guide*. Souvenir Press, 1977.
James, Duncan. *Antique Jewellery*. Shire, second edition 1998.
Launert, Edmund. *Scent and Scent Bottles*. Barrie & Jenkins, 1974.
Luthi, Ann Louise. *Sentimental Jewellery*. Shire, 1998; reprinted 2001.
Meredith, Alan and Gillian. *Buttons*. Shire, 2000; reprinted 2004.
Muller, Helen. *Jet Jewellery and Ornaments*. Shire, 1980; reprinted 2003.
Peacock, Primrose. *Buttons for the Collector*. David & Charles, 1972.
Sawdon, Mary. *A History of Victorian Skirt Grips*. Midsummer Books, 1995.
Walker, Alexandra. *Scent Bottles*. Shire, 1987; reprinted 2002.

Right: A full-length portrait of Annie Louisa Mary Lomax in 1908, showing the typical dress, hairstyle and hat of the Edwardian period.

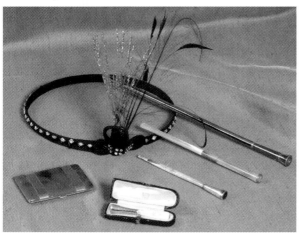

Left: *A collection of items typical of the 1920s. (Above) A 'flapper' head-dress, part original, of stiffened black velvet ribbon studded with diamanté stones and having a silvery centrepiece with black feathers. (Below, left to right) Smoking items: a slim brown cigarette case with silver banding; a small mother-of-pearl and silver cigarette holder in its original case; and three cigarette holders, one of bone with silver, one of mother-of-pearl, and a long painted wooden example.*

$\mathcal{P}$laces to visit

Before travelling, visitors should check the times and dates of opening of museums and also ascertain that relevant items are on show, as displays may be changed.

UNITED KINGDOM
Blaise Castle House Museum, Henbury Road, Henbury, Bristol BS10 7QS. Telephone: 0117 903 9818.
The British Museum, Great Russell Street, London WC1B 3DG. Telephone: 020 7323 8000 (switchboard); 020 7323 8299 (information desk). Website: www.thebritishmuseum.ac.uk
Cavalcade of Costume Museum, Lime Tree House, The Plocks, Blandford Forum, Dorset DT11 7AA. Telephone: 01258 453006.
Cecil Higgins Art Gallery, Castle Lane, The Embankment, Bedford MK40 3RP. Telephone: 01234 211222. Website: www.cecilhigginsartgallery.org
Chertsey Museum, The Cedars, 33 Windsor Street, Chertsey, Surrey KT16 8AT. Telephone: 01932 565764. Website: www.chertseymuseum.org.uk
The Fan Museum, 12 Crooms Hill, Greenwich, London SE10 8ER. Telephone: 020 8305 1441. Website: www.fan-museum.org
Fitzwilliam Museum, Trumpington Street, Cambridge CB2 1RB. Telephone: 01223 332900. Website: www.fitzmuseum.cam.ac.uk
Gallery of English Costume, Platt Hall, Platt Fields, Wilmslow Road, Rusholme, Manchester M14 5LL. Telephone: 0161 224 5217. Website: www.manchestergalleries.org
Hereford and Worcester County Museum, Hartlebury Castle, Hartlebury, Kidderminster, Worcestershire DY11 7XZ. Telephone: 01299 250416.
Killerton House (National Trust), Broadclyst, near Exeter, Devon EX5 3LE. Telephone: 01392 881345. Website: www.nationaltrust.org.uk

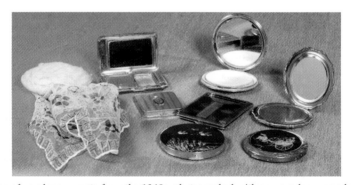

A collection of powder compacts from the 1940s, photographed with a swansdown powder puff in a fine silk handkerchief. (Left) The open, rectangular example is of brass, with a mirror in the lid, and is for powder and rouge; the square one below, a Stratnoid example, has an engine-turned decoration with a Royal Corps of Signals crest on the lid. (Centre, diagonally from top to bottom) A Stratton example, open to reveal mirror and powder puff over a gauze-covered powder container; a rectangular example, in typical Art Deco style, of imitation tortoiseshell with an elaborate scrolled-gilt decoration on the lid; a Stratnoid example, complete inside with gilt metal cover to the gauze-covered powder recess, the top decorated with ducks in flight over a lake with bulrushes. (Right) The open example has a brass cover for the powder container; the closed one below is decorated with a white rickshaw painting on a black background.

Two unusual purses, photographed with an exquisite mother-of-pearl snuff bottle and a fine aide-mémoire with mother-of-pearl covers. The purse on the left is cleverly made from small flat carved rectangular pieces of mother-of-pearl, expertly stitched together on a base of fabric, and is finished with a decorative edging; there are leather partitions inside. On the right is a purse made from angora rabbit fur, featuring a small animal's head with eyes, nose, mouth and teeth, a snap closure, and a white silk-cord handle.

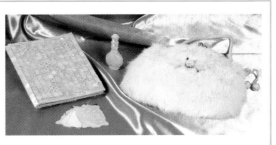

Museum of Costume, Assembly Rooms, Bennett Street, Bath BA1 2QH. Telephone: 01225 477789. Website: www.museumofcostume.co.uk
Museum of London, London Wall, London EC2Y 5HN. Telephone: 0870 444 3852. Website: www.museumoflondon.org.uk
Old House Museum, Cunningham Place, Bakewell, Derbyshire DE45 1DD. Telephone: 01629 813642.
The Stewartry Museum, 6 St Mary Street, Kirkcudbright, Scotland DG6 4AQ. Telephone: 01557 331643.
Victoria and Albert Museum, Cromwell Road, South Kensington, London SW7 2RL. Telephone: 020 7942 2000. Website: www.vam.ac.uk
Worthing Museum and Art Gallery, Chapel Road, Worthing, West Sussex BN11 1HP. Telephone: 01903 239999 extension 1140. Website: www.worthing.gov.uk
York Castle Museum, The Eye of York, York YO1 9RY. Telephone: 01904 650333. Website: www.yorkcastlemuseum.org.uk

NETHERLANDS
Tassenmuseum Hendrikje, Zonnestein 1, 1181 LR, Amstelveen, Netherlands. Telephone: (00 31) 2064 78681. Website: www.museumofbagsandpurses.com

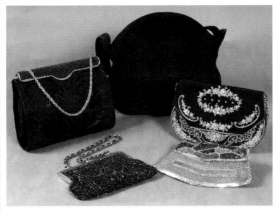

A group of bags and purses. (Clockwise from top left) Stiffened black grosgrain with top flap and gilt chain handle; soft, larger black grosgrain with matching handle; flower-embroidered black pochette with front flap and back wrist loop for security, lined with moiré fabric; typical Art Deco purse, the flap made from blue, red, green and gold sequins and the main part made from gold sequins with a strip of small gold rectangular ones edged with steel beads, and with a handle of silver-coloured beads stitched to a thread cord; small black-beaded bag on a silver-metal frame.

Index

Amber 20, 23
Amethyst 21, 25
Aquamarine 22
Art Deco 17, 21, 23, 51, 54
Art Nouveau 8, 25, 34, 51, 52
Arts and Crafts (Movement) 25, 51
Bakelite 16, 23, 33, 47
Bog-oak 20, 25
Brooches:
  bar 22
  regimental 6
  silver named 22
  sweetheart 6
Buckles 19, 26, 28
Butterfly 19, 22
Buttonhook 11, 29, 30, 36
Buttons 26, 27, 29
Cameo 8, 19
Card cases 12, 46
Chatelaine 11, 39, 40, 41
Chignon 8
Coral 8, 23
Crosses 19
Cymric 25
Czechoslovakia 17, 21, 23
Diamanté 23
Diamonds 19
Earrings 24
Ebony 7, 11
Edward VII, King 5
Edwardian 15, 23
Enamel 7, 33, 34
Faith, hope and charity 19
Fan 12, 49, 50, 51
First World War 5, 15, 51
Forget-me-not 19
French jet 1, 8, 9, 23, 25
Gilt 2, 6, 9, 12, 13, 19, 21, 23, 24
Glass 7, 14, 17
Glove powdering flask 36, 37
Glove stretchers 36, 37

Gloves 36, 37
Gold 18, 33, 35, 45
Goldstone 21, 24
Hair combs 8
Hair jewellery 21
Hallmark 10, 34, 41
Handbag 11, 39, 41
Hatpins 11, 32, 33, 34, 35
Hearts 23
Horseshoes 19
Insects 19
Ivory 21, 33, 37, 45
Jade 25
Jasper ware 12
Jet, French 1, 8, 9, 23, 25
Jet, Whitby 8, 21, 33
Jewellery 4, 8, 9, 18, 23
Limoges 8
Lockets 19, 21, 22
Lorgnette 12, 44, 45
Marcasite 22, 23
Mizpah 20, 22
Moonstone 22
Mosaic 1, 8
Mother of pearl 9, 10, 24, 33, 45, 46, 55
Necklaces, necklets 20, 23, 25
Nineteenth century 4, 5, 8, 13, 14, 18, 19, 21, 25, 26, 30, 40, 44, 45, 46, 51
Onyx 21, 24
Opals 19, 25
Parasol 12, 52
Paris backs 27
Paste 1, 23, 33
Peacock 22
Pearls 1, 19, 20, 21
Pendants 19, 22
Perfume 9, 13, 14, 16
Peridot 20, 22
Pinchbeck 45, 48
Piqué 8, 33, 45

Posé 8
Posy holder 12, 48
Powder compacts 42, 54
Prince Albert (Prince Consort) 5, 26
Prince of Wales feathers 21
Purses 39, 42, 43, 55
Purses, long 39, 40
Quizzing glasses 44, 45
Rhinestone 25
Ring stand 9, 11, 12
Rings 9
Salamander 22
Sapphire 20
Satsuma 27, 28, 33
Scent bottles 13, 14, 15, 16, 17.
Second World War 6, 7, 17
Sewing machine 5
Shells 19
Shoe horn 29, 30, 31
Silver 8, 9, 10, 29, 30, 33, 34, 35, 41, 45, 46
Skirt lifter 38, 41
Souvenirs 15, 22, 30, 34
Stars 19, 22
Steel 8, 21, 26, 33
Stickpins 12
Teddy bear 34
Tortoiseshell 8, 9, 21, 33, 45, 46
Tourmaline 22
Trifari 23, 25
Turquoise 1, 24, 25
Twentieth century 8, 9, 13, 19, 52
Victoria, Queen 5, 8, 21
Vinaigrette 14, 15
Vulcanite 25
Wedgwood 12
Worcester Royal Porcelain 8, 11, 14
Zip fastener 30, 43